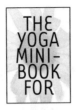

THE YOGA MINI-BOOK FOR

Longevity

A Specialized Program for a Healthier, Vital You

ELAINE GAVALAS

Illustrations by Nelle Davis

A Fireside Book · Published by Simon & Schuster · New York London Toronto Sydney Singapore

FIRESIDE
Rockefeller Center
1230 Avenue of the Americas
New York, NY 10020

For information regarding special discounts for bulk purchases, please contact
Simon & Schuster Special Sales at 1-800-456-6798 or business@simonandschuster.com

Designed by Chris Welch

Manufactured in the United States of America

1   3   5   7   9   10   8   6   4   2

Library of Congress Cataloging-in-Publication Data
Gavalas, Elaine.
The yoga minibook for longevity : a specialized program for a healthier,
vital you / Elaine Gavalas ; illustrations by Nelle Davis.
        p.   cm.
Includes index.
1. Longevity.   2. Yoga, Haòha.   I. Title.
            RA776.75 .G375   2003
613.7—dc21   2002030628

ISBN 0-7432-2699-2

DISCLAIMER

This publication contains the opinions and ideas of its author. It is intended to provide helpful and informative material on the subjects addressed in the publication. It is sold with the understanding that the author and publisher are not engaged in rendering medical, health, or any other kind of professional services in the book. The reader should consult his or her medical, health, or other competent professional before adopting any of the suggestions in this book or drawing inferences from it.

The author and publisher specifically disclaim all responsiblity for any liability, loss, or risk, personal or otherwise, which is incurred as a consequence, directly or indirectly, of the use and application of any of the contents of this book.

For my uncle, Arthur Vozeolas, and my Papous,
shining examples of graceful aging

Acknowledgments

This book would not have been possible without the help and creative contributions of my husband and writing guru, Stuart Katz. His brilliant literary judgment and patient work helped me bring this text to life. I am forever grateful for his extraordinary love, friendship, and support.

I wish to offer my heartfelt thanks to all of the talented professionals at Simon & Schuster Trade Paperbacks for producing my yoga minibook series, with special thanks to Trish Todd for providing me with the opportunity to write the books; to my editor, Lisa Considine, for her expertise and sage guidance; and to Anne Bartholomew, Martha Schwartz, and Janet Fletcher for their valuable assistance.

I also wish to extend my deepest gratitude and appreciation to my literary agent, Michael Psaltis (and the Ethan Ellenberg Literary Agency), for his wise counsel, encouragement, and support of my yoga books from the beginning.

I especially wish to thank Nelle Davis, who brought the yoga poses alive with her wonderful illustrations.

I am truly grateful to my parents-in-law, Ethel Katz Regolini and Leo Regolini, and my uncles, Arthur Vozeolas and Henry Kane, for their wisdom, help, and guidance.

Finally, many thanks to my yoga teachers (with special gratitude to Ram Dass), and to you, dear reader. May yoga bring you lasting health, happiness, peace, longevity, freedom, and bliss. *Om Shanthi* with love.

Contents

chapter 1

Understanding Yoga

Yoga for Longevity

Wouldn't you love to roll back the years and revive your youthful vigor and vitality? Perhaps your hope is to maintain your current fitness level for decades to come. Whether you're twenty-five, forty-five, or even sixty-five, you can turn to yoga for help.

The antiaging yoga program described in this book approaches lifelong wellness in a unique way that integrates the body, mind, and spirit. Regardless of how young or old you are, you'll find that practicing these poses for just a few minutes a day can turn back your biological clock and slow down most, if not all, of the declines associated with aging. Regular yoga practice is a wise investment in your physical and mental future from which you'll reap benefits well into your golden years.

The gentle stretching, strengthening, and soothing poses in Yoga for Longevity are suitable for people of all ages and all levels of fitness and flexibility. They're integrated into a lifestyle modification program that promotes longevity, reduces the risk of age-related diseases, and helps ease back problems, arthritis aches and pains, menopause and prostate problems, and diminished sexual drive or impotence.

You're never too old or too out of shape to begin a yoga program. After you've learned a few basic moves in Chapter 2, the real program begins with Chapter 3, "Easy Yoga," designed for absolute beginners, older adults, and people who haven't exercised in years. Don't be intimidated by the challenge of pretzel-like yoga poses so often featured in the press. Easy Yoga's simple postures will safely and gradually help you increase your workout intensity, whatever your starting point. Easy Yoga poses will also help improve and maintain your flexibility, aid in coordination and body control, increase your freedom of movement, and ultimately improve your balance.

From there you'll move on to the core of my longevity program, the Yoga Fountain of Youth. The dynamic combination of yoga and aerobics laid out in Chapter 4 promotes cardiovascular health, lowers the risk of cancer, strengthens muscles and bones, boosts immune system functioning, manages weight, and keeps skin looking young.

The chapter includes workouts at the Beginner, Intermediate, and Maintenance levels, and all of these workouts combine Sun Salutation and inversion poses.

You may be searching for a lasting fix for nagging back pain, or you may want to prevent future backaches. From a yoga point of view, overall wellness and longevity begin with a healthy spine. Practicing yoga poses from Chapter 5, "Yoga for a Youthful Back," just a few minutes a day is excellent insurance against back pain. With yoga-strengthened back muscles you'll be youthfully active for as long as you live.

If you're one of the millions of people who suffer from pain in their joints, Chapter 6, "Yoga to Relieve Aches and Pains," offers a soothing yoga practice to help ease and prevent such pain. Doing these yoga poses will help keep your joints and muscles supple, allowing you to move more easily. Yoga practice has been proven one of the most effective ways to restore joint health, relieve muscular tension, and improve strength.

The yoga poses offered in Chapter 7, "Yoga for Sex and Vitality," can help those experiencing unwelcome symptoms of perimenopause, menopause, osteoporosis, prostate problems, impotence, or reduced sex drive. Many detrimental midlife changes, such as diminishing hormone levels, weight gain, or loss of libido, can—at least in part—be alleviated by following this yoga program. In addition, the chapter includes a tantric yoga practice that can help you to enhance your sexuality.

I've found that combining yoga with self-massage and body-work techniques can be a powerful way to help restore the body's natural balance, increase well-being, and relieve chronic pain. In the chapters that follow you'll find yoga poses joined with self-massage techniques, such as *do-in* and self-acupressure. Together they will help to relieve and prevent tension and tightness, make your muscles more flexible, and increase your blood circulation.

Practiced together, yoga and self-massage are a dynamic healing duo. *Do-in* and acupressure are Asian self-massage healing techniques that have been practiced for thousands of years. Both employ touching, tapping, rubbing, applying pressure, and stretching to move the vital life force, called *ch'i* (or, in the yoga tradition, *prana*), to clear energy blockages, increase circulation, and harmonize the body. Self-massage balances ch'i vital energy with pressure and stretching of the acupressure points along meridian pathways through which ch'i flows. For many reasons, such as aging, illness, stress, and trauma, tension accumulates around the acupressure points, thereby obstructing the proper flow of ch'i through the body.

Self-massage helps release this tension so that your ch'i can circulate freely, optimizing your body's self-healing powers.

Another excellent way to complement and strengthen your yoga practice is to combine it with body-mind disciplines. Yoga for Longevity incorporates the Western somatic body-mind disciplines Ideokinesis and Pilates. These are therapeutic practices that retrain and integrate mind and body to improve movement efficiency. Ideokinesis is a system of movement education and therapy based on the use of visualization and imagery. In Chapter 5, you'll learn how to use Ideokinesis imagery as you practice specific yoga poses to reeducate and integrate your body's movement patterns. The Pilates method is a system of body conditioning and strengthening exercises focused on the abdominal, pelvic, and back muscles—the "power center," or "core," of the body. Also in Chapter 5, specialized Pilates movements are incorporated into yoga poses to help you build "core" strength (without building bulk) and improve your alignment and flexibility.

Over the years, I have studied and practiced many hatha yoga styles, such as Integral, Iyengar, ashtanga vinyasa, kundalini, mantra, raja, and tantra, and have been especially interested in yoga's therapeutic applications. I have observed individuals and groups practicing yoga, and have seen its power to help them lose weight and relieve stress while they increase their energy, strength, and longevity. I've written my yoga minibook series—the first four being *The Yoga Minibook for Weight Loss, The Yoga Minibook for Longevity, The Yoga Minibook for Stress Relief,* and *The Yoga Minibook for Energy and Strength*—as self-help guides in response to people's many fitness, diet, and wellness problems, questions, and concerns. I've had an opportunity to apply yoga techniques to help people achieve their wellness goals, and I've seen spectacular results.

My greatest wish is to share with you the many wonderful benefits yoga practice has given to me and the individuals I've assisted over the years. Whether you're looking to lose weight, boost your energy, relieve stress, or find the fountain of youth, I've created a yoga book for you.

But before we dive in, a little background.

21st Century Yoga

Throughout the centuries, yoga has redefined and re-created itself to meet the needs of different eras and cultures. Yoga was barely known in the Western world until the 1960s, when the Beatles went off to India to find spiritual enlightenment with Maharishi Mahesh Yogi. Since then, yoga has evolved from a practice for hippie spiritual seekers chanting *om* with Swami Ṣatchidananda at Woodstock in 1969 to a practice embraced by everyone from Hollywood stars striving for beautiful bodies and high-powered CEOs seeking stress relief, to baby boomers wanting to turn back the hands of time. Even United States Supreme Court Justice Sandra Day O'Connor takes a weekly yoga class. At least fifteen million Americans include some form of yoga in their fitness regimen.

Although yoga has been celebrated as the new fitness philosophy for the twenty-first century, the practice of yoga actually goes back thousands of years. Yoga originated in India and is an ancient philosophical discipline, not a religion. Originally yoga was practiced as a path to spiritual enlightenment, a way of arriving at a state of pure bliss and oneness with the universe. *Yoga* is a Sanskrit word meaning "union"; it describes the integration of body, mind, and spirit, and communion with a universal energy, the Supreme Consciousness. The practice of hatha yoga, whose exercises are familiar to many Westerners, was originally devised to strengthen the body and prepare it for the long, motionless hours of meditation.

Yoga dates back to the ancient Vedas, sacred Hindu scriptures first recorded around 2500 B.C.E. Over millennia, the yoga tradition has evolved into eight principal branches, which are different paths that all lead to the same goal: enlightenment.

The eight branches of yoga are called the Wheel of Yoga. They are:

Hatha Yoga (pronounced *haht-ha*), the yoga of physical discipline and bodily mastery. This is the branch of yoga most of us in the West are familiar with, and it is the one presented in this book. In hatha, enlightenment is achieved through spiritualized physical practices including *asanas* (postures), *pranayama* (controlled breathing), and meditation. The *Hatha Yoga Pradipika*, a fourteenth-century text, is a guide to hatha yoga.

Jhana Yoga (pronounced *gyah-nah*), the yoga of wisdom and knowledge. In jhana, enlightenment and self-realization are achieved through the teaching of nondualism, the elimination of illusion, and direct knowledge of the divine.

Bhakti Yoga (pronounced *bhuk-tee*), the path to achieve union with the divine through love and acts of devotion.

Karma Yoga (pronounced *kahr-mah*), the path of enlightenment through selfless service and actions.

Mantra Yoga (pronounced *mahn-trah*), the yoga of sacred sounds for self-awakening. A form of mantra yoga familiar to Westerners is Transcendental Meditation (TM).

Kundalini Yoga (pronounced *koon-da-lee-nee*), the activation of the latent spiritual energy stored in the body and raised along the spine to the head through the breath and movement.

Tantra Yoga (pronounced *tahn-trah*), union with all that you are, achieved by harnessing sexual energy. Although tantra yoga has become famous for some rituals that spiritualize sexuality, it is essentially a spiritual discipline of nonsexual rituals and visualizations that activate spiritual energy.

Raja Yoga (pronounced *rah-jah*)—also known as royal, classical, eight-limbed, or ashtanga (not to be confused with the separate ashtanga style of yoga)—yoga of the mind and mental mastery. In the second century B.C.E., the great Hindu sage Patanjali wrote down the principles of classical yoga in the *Yoga Sutras.* Patanjali describes eight steps, or "limbs," known as the Tree of Yoga. These eight limbs provide ethical guidelines for living and help along the yoga path to enlightenment.

The Tree of Yoga is composed of

Yama (pronounced *yah-mah*), the roots of the tree, which are moral discipline and ethical restraints. These include nonviolence (*ahimsa*), truthfulness, freedom from avarice, chastity, and noncovetousness.

Niyama (pronounced *nee-yah-mah*), the trunk of the tree, which represents self-restraint and observance, including cleanliness, contentment, self-discipline, introspection or self-study, and devotion.

Asana (pronounced *ah-sah-nah*), the branches of the tree. It includes the postures of hatha yoga.

Pranayama (pronounced *prah-nah-yah-mah*), the leaves of the tree. It includes breath control for circulation of *prana,* or life-force energy.

Pratyahara (pronounced *prah-tyah-hah-rah*), the bark of the tree. It includes withdrawal of the senses for meditation.

Dharana (pronounced *dah-rah-nah*), the sap. It includes concentration for meditation.

Dhyana (pronounced *dee-yah-nah*), the flower. It includes meditation.

Samadhi (pronounced *sah-mah-dhee*), the fruit. It is the state of pure consciousness, or total bliss. All of the limbs of yoga lead to samadhi.

Your Yoga Practice

Whether you're nine or ninety, you can enjoy and greatly benefit from practicing yoga. Its requirements are minimal. You need only

30 to 60 minutes each day; a nonskid mat; comfortable, nonrestrictive clothing; and a small exercise space. Turn off your phone, put on the answering machine, and let your family and friends know that you're not to be disturbed during your yoga time—unless, of course, they want to join you.

You'll notice that the practice workouts in this book include poses that stretch the spine in six directions. In yoga there is a saying, "You're as young as your spine." If you stretch your spine in six directions during your daily practice you will be richly rewarded with a youthful, flexible, strong back and body. The six directions (and some representative postures) are:

- Forward (Standing Forward Bend)
- Backward (Standing Backbend)
- Right side (Seated Side-to-Side Right)
- Left side (Seated Side-to-Side Left)
- Right twist (Seated Twist Right)
- Left twist (Seated Twist Left)

Every yoga workout ends with a Relaxation period (see Chapter 2, "Before You Begin"). As you progress in your yoga study, you will also want to add meditation and breathing exercises (see Chapter 2). As I mentioned earlier, yoga is a noncompetitive practice. There's no need to compete with other yogis or yoginis. Simply do the best that you can each and every time you practice. Your body will respond differently to the postures from day to day because of various factors, such as your diet, the amount of sleep you've had, and the time of day you're practicing. It is important to remember that the practice of yoga is a journey and an exploration into the nature of your self.

Practicing yoga is well worth it. If you're interested in a lifetime of radiantly good health and sexual vitality, then this is the book for you. *Namaste!* (*Namaste* is a traditional yoga blessing that means "The divine in me bows to the divine in you.")

Your Yoga for Longevity Program

The Yoga for Longevity Program includes five workout steps for maximizing longevity benefits in the shortest time possible. Begin with Step 1 and continue with Steps 2 through 5, according to your physical condition and capabilities. An overview of the steps and workout plans follows. You can find a more detailed description of each workout plan in Chapters 2 through 7.

Step 1: Basics and Easy Yoga Workout

Step 2: Yoga Fountain of Youth Workout Plans (including

Beginner, Intermediate, and Maintenance Yoga
Fountain of Youth Workouts)

Step 3: Yoga Back Workout

Step 4: 10-Minute Yoga Relief Workout

Step 5: Yoga for Sexual Vitality Workout

STEP 1. BASICS AND EASY YOGA WORKOUT

Begin with the Yoga Basics and Easy Yoga poses found in Chapters 2 and 3, and practice for 2 weeks. Do these poses for 30 to 40 minutes, 3 or 4 days a week. Each practice session includes Warm Up with Yoga Basics poses, Easy Yoga postures practice, and a Cool Down/Relaxation period with a few more Basics poses. Be aware that it may take you more than 2 weeks to do this routine comfortably, depending on your physical condition. If you feel comfortable and confident doing these poses, proceed to the Yoga Fountain of Youth Workouts found in Chapter 4. Otherwise, stay with Weeks 1 and 2 until you feel strong enough to continue. See Chapters 2 and 3 for the poses and detailed workout.

STEP 2. YOGA FOUNTAIN OF YOUTH WORKOUTS

Following 2 weeks of Yoga Basics and Easy Yoga, begin on the 4-week Yoga Fountain of Youth Workouts (Beginner, Intermediate, and Maintenance) found in Chapter 4. These workouts will help you reach your longevity goals in the shortest time possible. Each practice session includes Warm Up, Sun Salutation, inversion poses, and a Cool Down/Relaxation period. As you progress from Beginner to Maintenance over a period of months, you'll build your yoga practice up from 30 to 60 minutes a day, 3 to 5 days a week. See Chapter 4 for the detailed workouts.

For additional longevity benefits, you can incorporate the Yoga Back Workout, the 10-Minute Yoga Relief Workout, or the Yoga for Sexual Vitality Workout into your practice (see Chapters 5, 6, and 7).

1. Beginner Fountain of Youth Workout
Weeks 1 Through 4

Start with the Beginners Fountain of Youth Workout, combining Sun Salutation and inversion poses, for 30 to 40 minutes, 3 days a week. Be aware that it may take you more than 4 weeks to do this routine comfortably, depending on your physical condition.

2. Intermediate Fountain of Youth Workout
Weeks 1 through 4

After completing the Beginner Fountain of Youth Workout, continue with the Intermediate Fountain of Youth Workout, combining Sun Salutation and inversion poses for 40 minutes, 4 or 5 days a week. Be aware that it may take you more than 4 weeks to do this routine comfortably, depending on your physical condition.

3. Maintenance Fountain of Youth Workout
Week 1 and Beyond

After completing the Intermediate Yoga Fountain of Youth Workout, continue with the Maintenance Fountain of Youth Workout, combining Sun Salutation and inversion poses, for 40 minutes, 5 days a week.

STEP 3. YOGA BACK WORKOUT

This 4-week yoga program for your back can be practiced alone or in conjunction with the Yoga Fountain of Youth Workouts. Do these poses for 15 to 20 minutes a day, 3 days a week. Be aware that it may take you more than 4 weeks to do this routine comfortably, depending on your physical condition. See Chapter 5 for the detailed workout.

STEP 4. 10-MINUTE YOGA RELIEF WORKOUT

This 4-week yoga program for relief from aches and pains can be practiced alone or combined with the Yoga Fountain of Youth Workouts. Do these poses for 10 minutes, 3 days a week. Be aware that it may take you more than 4 weeks to do this routine comfortably, depending on your physical condition. See Chapter 6 for the detailed workout.

STEP 5. YOGA FOR SEXUAL VITALITY WORKOUT

This 4-week yoga program for sexual vitality can be practiced alone or combined with the Yoga Fountain of Youth Workouts. Do these poses for 10 to 15 minutes, 3 days a week. Be aware that it may take you more than 4 weeks to do this routine comfortably, depending on your physical condition. See Chapter 7 for the detailed workout.

Before You Begin

Before you begin your Yoga for Longevity Program, you should heed the following cautions, as well as set some realistic goals. You can then begin your longevity program with the Yoga Basics and Easy Yoga Program, which is laid out in this chapter and the one that follows.

A Word of Caution

Yoga should never cause you pain. Due to the intense stretching in some of the yoga poses, you need to be tuned in to your body. You should be aware of and realistic about where your "edge"—the point beyond which your body can't comfortably go any further—is in each pose. Being at your edge should never cause a burning feeling of pain. As you explore each yoga pose, go slowly and cautiously, finding the point to which you can stretch safely. As you gradually become stronger and more flexible, you'll find that your edge will change. You'll be able comfortably and safely to stretch further and hold the poses longer.

Before beginning any new exercise program, you should always consult your health care practitioner, especially if you have health problems or physical limitations. Also, women should be aware that practicing inverted postures, such as Supported Shoulderstand with Wall and Legs-up-the-Wall Pose, are not recommended during the first few days of menstruation. If you are pregnant, be sure to obtain clearance from your physician before beginning a hatha yoga program. There are many excellent prenatal yoga classes with certified instructors that teach specific prenatal yoga routines.

Never practice yoga poses that cause you pain or discomfort. If pain persists, be sure to consult your health care professional.

Your Longevity Goals

Before beginning your yoga practice, try to be clear about your goals. How much time are you allowing yourself to reach your antiaging and fitness goals? Set reasonable goals and know that it will take some time to reach them. Starting with your first yoga lesson, you'll begin to turn back your biological clock. However, it usually takes a minimum of 2 to 3 months of consistent yoga practice to build up healthful habits that help slow the declines associated with aging.

It also takes a minimum of 2 to 3 months of consistent yoga exercise before changes in strength, flexibility, and body composition (less fat and more muscle) begin to appear. Depending on your physical condition when you begin this yoga program, it may even be 6 months or more before your body really starts to show results. Rest assured, though, correct, consistent practice will result in positive changes. You may want to begin a yoga journal and jot down your thoughts about how you look and feel, to help you pinpoint areas you would like to change.

It's a good idea to check your progress every month or two and reevaluate your goals. For example, after 6 weeks you may be finishing the Beginner Yoga Fountain of Youth Workout (in Chapter 4). At this point, you will want to determine your progress, consider what types of physical challenges you may be experiencing, and perhaps establish a new set of goals. Depending on these results, you may want to progress to the Intermediate Yoga Fountain of Youth Workout and incorporate the Yoga Back Workout, or the 10-Minute Yoga Relief Workout, or the Yoga for Sexual Vitality Workout into your practice for additional longevity benefits. Or you may decide to continue practicing the Beginner Yoga Fountain of Youth Workout without any add-ons for a while longer.

Please keep in mind that this yoga antiaging plan is not only a workout, it's a lifestyle modification program that will build healthful habits to promote longevity and improve and protect the quality of your health and appearance. Make a daily affirmation to yourself to reach your antiaging goals through consistent yoga exercise and breathing and meditation practice.

Yoga Basics

An understanding of certain fundamental movements will help you perform the yoga postures in this book correctly. These movements are incorporated into many yoga postures and will help you build strength, flexibility, and proper alignment in your upper body and lower back.

The squeeze, hold, and release actions found in Shoulder Press and Squeeze and Pelvic Tilt are fundamental to yoga practice, massaging tension and stress out of a particular area while bringing fresh, oxygenated blood to the muscles and tissues. The lifting-the-sternum action found in Mountain Pose is repeated over and over again within many yoga postures.

The use of your core strength—the lifting of your abdominal muscles for maximum support—is also essential while performing yoga postures. In yoga, this includes the *mula bandha*, or "root lock," which contracts the perineum, and the *uddiyana bandha*, which contracts the abdomen. The mula bandha (see page 30) and uddiyana bandha (see Easy Stomach Lift, page 54) actions are incorporated into the yoga poses and draw awareness to the core of your body, building a strong foundation in your abdominal, pelvic, and genital muscles.

Ujjayi breathing is a classic yoga breathing technique that is practiced while holding poses (see Ujjayi Pranayama, page 30). It is combined with Sun Salutation (see Chapter 4) to link the postures together and promote concentration, calm, and meditation. Supported Relaxation should be included at the end of your yoga session whenever possible, to calm your mind and nervous system.

Basics and Easy Yoga Workout

Begin your first 2 weeks of yoga practice with the Yoga Basics poses that follow and the Easy Yoga poses from Chapter 3. Be aware that it may take you more than 2 weeks to do this routine comfortably, depending on your physical condition. If you feel comfortable and confident doing these poses, proceed to the Yoga Fountain of Youth Workout found in Chapter 4. Otherwise, stay with Weeks 1 and 2 until you feel strong enough to continue.

Week 1

Workout Schedule: Practice for 30 minutes, 3 times a week. Warm Up with Yoga Basics poses, proceed to Easy Yoga poses, and then Cool Down with a few more Yoga Basics poses.

Warm Up:
Shoulder Press and Squeeze
Mountain Pose and Lifting the Sternum
Pelvic Tilt
Chest Expander

Easy Yoga:

Seated Shoulder Rolls

Seated Side-to-Side

Seated Wheel Pose

Seated Forward Bend in Chair

Seated Twist

Seated Leg Lifts

Seated Eye Yoga

Cool Down:

Mula Bandha

Complete Breath

Seated Relaxation Pose with Yoga Observation Meditation

Week 2

Workout Schedule: Practice for 30 to 40 minutes, 4 times a week. Warm Up with Yoga Basics poses, proceed to Easy Yoga poses, and then Cool Down with a few more Yoga Basics poses.

Warm Up:

Shoulder Press and Squeeze

Mountain Pose and Lifting the Sternum

Pelvic Tilt

Chest Expander

Easy Yoga:

Downward-Facing Dog with Chair

Upward-Facing Dog with Chair

Modified Tree Pose

Modified Warrior III

Easy Stomach Lift

Modified Dancer Pose

Modified Chair Pose

Cool Down:

Mula Bandha

Ujjayi Pranayama

Supported Relaxation Pose with Yoga Observation Meditation

Yoga Basics Poses

SHOULDER PRESS AND SQUEEZE

What It Does. These shoulder movements are incorporated into many yoga postures, including Cobra Pose, Downward-Facing

Dog, and Dolphin Headstand Preparation. These squeeze, hold, and release actions are fundamental to yoga practice, massaging tension and stress out of a particular area while bringing fresh, oxygenated blood into the muscles and tissues.

How to Do It:

1. Sit up straight on the mat with your legs crossed, arms at your sides.

2. Inhale and raise your shoulders toward your ears. Squeeze and hold for 4 counts. Exhale and release, pressing your shoulders down and away from your ears.

3. Clasp your hands behind your back. Inhale and straighten your elbows. Press your shoulders down, away from your ears. Exhale and gently squeeze your shoulder blades together. Hold for 3 counts. Release your hands.

4. Repeat.

MOUNTAIN POSE AND LIFTING THE STERNUM (TADASANA)

What It Does: The subtle but important action of lifting the sternum or breastbone toward the ceiling is incorporated into many yoga postures, including Standing Backbend and Modified Head-to-Knee Pose.

How to Do It:

1. Stand in Mountain Pose, feet together, legs straight, and hands in prayer position over your heart center. Visualize a string attached to your sternum, or breastbone (the bone in the center of your chest).

2. Inhale and visualize the string being pulled up toward the ceiling. Feel the subtle lifting and expanding of your chest, rib cage, and sternum, lengthening the front of your body. Keep your shoulders relaxed and down, away from your ears.

3. Exhale and release.

4. Repeat.

PELVIC TILT IN MODIFIED RELAXATION POSE
(MODIFIED SAVASANA)

What It Does: These pelvic movements are incorporated into many yoga postures, including Standing Backbend and Bridge 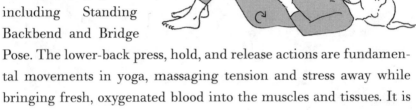 Pose. The lower-back press, hold, and release actions are fundamental movements in yoga, massaging tension and stress away while bringing fresh, oxygenated blood into the muscles and tissues. It is essential to tighten the buttock muscles firmly to protect and stabilize your lower back and activate the abdominals.

How to Do It:

1. Lie on your back on the mat, knees bent and feet flat to the mat, hip-width apart. Rest your hands on your abdomen. Inhale and allow your lower back to arch naturally.

2. Exhale, tightening your buttock muscles, tilting your pelvis under, and pulling your abdomen in. Press the small of your back gently to the mat. Inhale and release.

3. Repeat the exercise.

CHEST EXPANDER

What it Does: This exercise incorporates elements of all three movements that came before: the Shoulder Press and Squeeze, Mountain Pose and Lifting the Sternum, and Pelvic Tilt. If your shoulders and chest are tight, try clasping a towel or belt behind you while doing this exercise.

How to Do It:

1. Stand with your feet hip-width apart and clasp your hands behind your back.

2. Inhale, lifting your sternum toward the ceiling as you press your shoulders down and away from your ears. Exhale, straightening your elbows and gently squeezing your shoulder blades together. Tighten the buttock muscles, tilt the pelvis under, and pull the abdomen in.

3. Inhale, release, and relax.

COMPLETE BREATH (PRANAYAMA)

What It Does: Research indicates that breathing slowly and deeply sends a message to the body and mind that all is well, thereby interrupting the stress cycle. Deep, diaphragmatic breathing requires all of the abdominal muscles to compress and expel the air from the lungs completely.

How to Do It:

1. Sit comfortably in a chair, or on the floor in a cross-legged position. Keep your back straight and your neck and head aligned with your spinal column.

2. Breathe in slowly through your nose (mouth closed!) to the count of 4. Allow your diaphragm to descend, expanding the middle rib cage, then expanding the base of the lungs. Hold for a moment.

3. Breathe out through your nose, releasing the air slowly to the count of 8. Exhale from the upper part of the lungs, then the middle rib cage. Slightly contract your abdominal muscles and squeeze all the air out.

4. Repeat 6 times.

UJJAYI PRANAYAMA

What It Does: Ujjayi breathing is a classic pranayama (yoga breathing) technique that is practiced while holding poses, and is combined with Sun Salutation to link the postures together and promote concentration, calm, and meditation.

How to Do It:

1. Keeping your lips closed, constrict the back of your throat, or the glottis (the opening between the vocal chords), during inhalation and exhalation. This produces a hissing sound, like that heard at the approach of Darth Vader.

2. If this is too difficult, start by whispering the sound *aaah* while inhaling and exhaling through your open mouth.

3. Then close your lips and breathe through your nose, continuing to make the hissing *aaah* sound at the back of your throat.

MULA BANDHA

What It Does: The mula bandha, or "root lock," contracts the perineum, or pelvic floor, which comprises the pubococcygeus muscles between the rectum and genitals. This draws awareness to the core of your body, strengthening the abdominal, pelvic, and genital muscles.

How to Do It:

1. Sit straight and tall on a chair or cross-legged on the floor. To visualize where your pelvic muscles are, imagine stopping the flow of your urine. Inhale, then exhale and contract these muscles, pulling up through your genital area and drawing up through your spine. Inhale and release the muscles.

2. Isolate the muscle group around your anus. Inhale, then exhale, contracting the muscles and drawing them upward. Inhale and release the muscles.

3. Now combine the two actions. Inhale, then exhale and contract the muscles of your anus and genitals at the same time. Inhale and release the muscles.

SUPPORTED RELAXATION POSE *(SUPPORTED SAVASANA)*

What It Does: It enhances the effectiveness of the poses, calms the mind and nervous system, and helps relieve insomnia. End your yoga practice with this pose.

How to Do It:

1. Lie on your back on a mat on the floor with a folded blanket under your head and neck. You may want to put an additional folded blanket or two under your back.

2. Place your feet a comfortable distance apart. The hands are at the sides, palms turned upward. Move your shoulders down, away from your ears, and tuck your shoulder blades in toward your spine. If your back feels uncom- 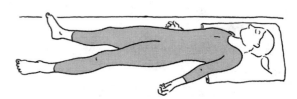 fortable, bend your knees as much as you need to, to alleviate pain or discomfort. You may feel more comfortable with a folded blanket or a pillow underneath your knees.

3. Inhale. Exhale, contracting the buttock muscles and pressing the curve out of your lower back. Release and relax completely.

4. Relax each part of your body. Begin by focusing your attention on your feet and toes. Inhale and suggest to your feet and toes that they relax. Exhale and feel your feet and toes relaxing. Repeat this relaxation procedure with each individual body part.

5. Practice Yoga Observation Meditation (see below).

6. Relax all efforts and rest in the stillness for as long as you wish.

YOGA OBSERVATION MEDITATION

What It Does: Yoga Observation Meditation practices *svadhyaya* (the understanding of self), which is part of niyama, one of the eight limbs of yoga as described in Patanjali's *Yoga Sutras* (see Chapter 1). This practice includes self-observation, which nurtures introspection, serenity, and cosmic connectedness, ultimately leading to a universal union with all that you are.

How to Do It:

1. Sit straight on a chair with your legs together and feet flat on the floor, or lie down in Supported Relaxation Pose. Be sure that you're comfortable and relaxed in this position.

2. For several minutes or longer, sense the changes going on in your body externally and internally. Observe how you're feeling. How does your skin feel? Does it tingle? Is it warm? After your yoga stretches, sense and enjoy the energy and warmth flowing to areas that were previously stiff with tension or fatigue. Consciously try to relax any areas that are still tense, fatigued, or painful.

3. Calmly take note of the flow of your thoughts. Is your mind restless? Do you have negative thoughts and suggestions? Quiet your mind by focusing on your breath. Center your attention on the tip of your nose. Observe the coolness of the air as it flows into your nostrils, and the warmth of the air as it flows out. Hold your attention on your breath. If your mind wanders, simply bring it back to the breath as it flows in and out of your nostrils. Be in the moment.

4. Now replace your negative thoughts with positive suggestions, such as uplifting words, affirmations, thoughts, and prayers. Breathe in love, light, energy, and healing to every cell of your body. Breathe out all negativity, darkness, tension, and fatigue. Rest your body and mind for as long as you like.

Easy Yoga

D o you think you're too old or out of shape to begin a yoga program? Put that misguided notion to rest. It's never too late to start exercising with yoga. Yoga practice doesn't have to be strenuous for you to derive and enjoy all its benefits. No matter your age, size, shape, or fitness level, the Easy Yoga routine described in this chapter will help you maintain your vitality, boost your immunity, and keep you fit. Whether you're an absolute beginner or haven't exercised in years, starting with this workout will build your strength, stamina, and confidence without injury or strain. Easy Yoga will teach you how to work within your fitness zone and respect your own level of ability.

Yoga isn't just for young, ultraflexible people, although the media often portray it that way. On the contrary, yoga's greatest benefits are for those who need it the most. Older adults, beginners, or individuals recovering from an illness may be intimidated by pictures of advanced practitioners in pretzel-like poses. The reality is that many of these exercises are simple and can be done sitting on a chair, couch, or bed. Regardless of your age and fitness level at the start, you can safely and gradually increase the intensity of your yoga workouts to reach your antiaging and fitness goals.

One of the most important indicators of overall fitness and youthfulness is good balance, which commonly diminishes over time. In older adults, this loss of balance and flexibility can lead to dangerous falls and devastating accidents. A traumatic fall can trigger a series of events that ultimately limit the individual's mobility and freedom. The good news is that studies have shown that low- and moderate-intensity exercise, such as this Easy Yoga workout, can improve your balance and prevent falls. By exercising, even people in their eighties and nineties have regained lost range of motion and pain-free movement.

Chair Yoga

Yoga can be modified for anyone who has difficulty balancing, or has limited flexibility, tight joints, or almost any other physical challenge. If you have difficulty lying or sitting on the floor, Easy Yoga can be done on a chair or on the edge of a bed. You can derive the same benefits you would from classic yoga poses with the modified chair poses that you'll find in this chapter.

Proceed through the workout slowly, safely, and with awareness. Work the poses at your comfort level. Don't ever strain or force your body to the point of pain. The practice of yoga is the antithesis of the no-pain, no-gain approach to working out.

Modify the Poses

Once you're comfortable with chair yoga and you begin to gain strength and flexibility, you'll want to progress to the next level by modifying your yoga poses with props, such as a wall, a bolster, a belt or strap, blankets, blocks, and pillows. These props help compensate for physical limitations, such as difficulty reaching your arms above your head or sitting on the floor. Using props will help prevent muscle, back, and knee strain due to weakness, lack of flexibility, and balance problems.

Standing postures and inverted poses can present a challenge for beginners of any age. The standing poses found in this chapter, such as Modified Tree Pose, Modified Chair Pose, Modified Warrior III,

Easy Stomach Lift, and Modified Dancer Pose, develop balance and strength and can be safely practiced with a chair or wall for support. Inversion poses, such as headstands and shoulderstands, can increase the risk of spinal injury and should be avoided, but you can still derive the benefits of an inverted pose with a combination of Downward-Facing Dog with Chair and Upward-Facing Dog with Chair.

As you progress, you will naturally want to add the more challenging workouts in Chapter 4. By gradually adding more difficult poses to your practice and modifying the poses with props as needed, you will soon find your body becoming stronger and more flexible, as you grow calmer, more confident, and more optimistic.

Basics and Easy Yoga Workout

No matter what your age or fitness level, begin your first 2 weeks of yoga practice with the Easy Yoga poses that follow and the Yoga Basics poses from Chapter 2. Be aware that it may take you more than 2 weeks to do this routine comfortably, depending on your physical condition. If you feel comfortable and confident doing these poses, proceed to the Yoga Fountain of Youth Workouts found in Chapter 4.

Otherwise, stay with Weeks 1 and 2 until you feel strong enough to continue.

Week 1

Workout Schedule: Practice for 30 minutes, 3 times a week. Warm Up with Yoga Basics poses, proceed to Easy Yoga poses, and then Cool Down with a few more Yoga Basics poses.

Warm Up:

Shoulder Press and Squeeze

Mountain Pose and Lifting the Sternum

Pelvic Tilt

Chest Expander

Easy Yoga:

Seated Shoulder Rolls

Seated Side-to-Side

Seated Wheel Pose

Seated Forward Bend in Chair

Seated Twist

Seated Leg Lifts

Seated Eye Yoga

Cool Down:

Mula Bandha

Complete Breath

Seated Relaxation Pose with Yoga Observation Meditation

Week 2

Workout Schedule: Practice for 30 to 40 minutes, 4 times a week. Warm Up with Yoga Basics poses, proceed to Easy Yoga poses, and then Cool Down with a few more Yoga Basics poses.

Warm Up:

Shoulder Press and Squeeze

Mountain Pose and Lifting the Sternum

Pelvic Tilt

Chest Expander

Easy Yoga:

Downward-Facing Dog with Chair

Upward-Facing Dog with chair

Modified Tree Pose

Modified Warrior III

Easy Stomach Lift

Modified Dancer Pose

Modified Chair Pose

Cool Down:

Mula Bandha

Ujjayi Pranayama

Supported Relaxation Pose with Yoga Observation Meditation

Easy Yoga Asanas

SEATED SHOULDER ROLLS

What It Does: Releases tension and fatigue in the neck, shoulders, and upper back.

How to Do It:

1. Sit straight in a chair with your legs together and feet flat on the floor. Inhale as you slowly lift both your shoulders toward your ears. Exhale as you release your shoulders. Repeat 3 times.

2. Rotate your shoulders in a circle, lifting them toward your ears, then rolling them back, down, forward, and up. Repeat 2 times.

3. Now reverse the shoulder roll, lifting both your shoulders toward your ears, then rolling them forward, down, back, and up. Repeat 2 times and then relax your shoulders.

SEATED SIDE-TO-SIDE *(MODIFIED NITAMBASANA)*

What It Does: It releases tension and fatigue in the upper body and helps relieve lower-back tightness.

How to Do It:

1. Sit straight on a chair with your feet flat on the floor. Inhale, raising your arms up behind your ears, your palms facing each other. Stretch your torso and rib cage upward.

2. Exhale, stretching to the right. Pull your abdomen in. Look under your left arm. Inhale as you return to center. Repeat left.

3. Lower your arms and come to a relaxed seated position.

SEATED WHEEL POSE *(MODIFIED CHAKRASANA)*

What It Does: It increases spinal flexibility, improves breathing, tones the internal organs, and improves posture.

How to Do It:

1. Sit straight at the edge of your chair with feet flat on the floor, hands resting on the arm-rests or lightly on the seat of the chair.

2. Inhale and arch, lifting your breast-bone. Lift your chin and gaze upward. Do not crunch your neck as you bring your chin up; bring your head back only as far as you can support it. Hold for 3 breaths.

3. Release to a relaxed seated position.

SEATED FORWARD BEND IN CHAIR *(MODIFIED UTTANASANA)*

What It Does: It stretches the back, tones the abdominals, calms the nerves, and quiets the mind. As you build strength, practice Modified Spread-Leg Forward Bend (see page 115).

How to Do It:

1. Sit straight on a chair with your legs together and feet flat on the floor.

2. Inhale. Exhale, rounding your shoulders and spine forward, one vertebra at a time. Lower your forehead to your knees, laying chest on thighs as your arms hang down by your legs. Feel your back and shoulder muscles stretch as you relax in the position for 3 breaths.

3. Place your hands on your knees and slowly roll up, one vertebra at a time, raising your head last. Repeat.

SEATED TWIST (MODIFIED BHARADVAJASANA)

What It Does: It increases spine and neck flexibility, and it releases tension and fatigue from the back muscles.

How to Do It:

1. Sit straight in a chair with your legs together and feet flat on the floor. Inhale, lengthen your spine, and place your left hand on your right knee and your right hand on the back of the chair.

2. Exhale and gently twist your body right, turning your belly, then your chest, then your shoulders, then your head, directing your gaze over your right shoulder. Keep your shoulder blades down and in. Hold for 3 breaths.

3. Slowly return to center, beginning with the belly, then the chest, shoulder, head, and eyes.

4. Repeat the twist to the left.

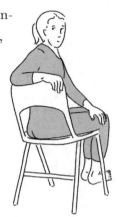

SEATED LEG LIFTS

What It Does: It stretches and strengthens the legs and hips.

How to Do It:

1. Sit straight on a chair with your legs together and feet flat on the floor. Lightly hold the sides of your chair. Inhale as you straighten your right leg and raise it. Pull the kneecap up so the thigh muscles feel firm. Hold for 4 seconds.

2. Exhale as you lower the right leg to the floor.

3. Repeat with your left leg.

4. Repeat once on each side, building up to 5 times.

SEATED EYE YOGA

What It Does: Yoga eye exercises will help maintain the strength and health of your eyes as well as prevent eyestrain and tiredness. Do this exercise gradually; do not overtire or strain your eyes.

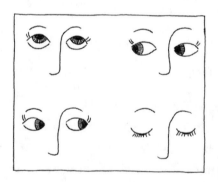

How to Do It:

1. Sit comfortably in a chair with your feet flat on the floor. If you're wearing eyeglasses, be sure to remove them. Circle your eyes slowly in a clockwise direction. Raise your eyes up toward the ceiling, move them to the right as far as possible, then down to the floor, and then to the left, as far as possible. There should be no strain or pain while doing this.

2. Repeat the complete circle with your eyes in the opposite (counterclockwise) direction.

3. Repeat each complete circle (clockwise, then counterclockwise) once.

4. Now rest and relax your eyes. Rub your hands together vigorously to warm them. Place your palms lightly over your eyes for a minute. Next, with your fingertips, gently massage around your eyes and along your cheekbones.

SEATED RELAXATION POSE *(MODIFIED SAVASANA)*

What It Does: Always end your yoga practice with a Relaxation Pose. This will enhance the effectiveness of all that's come before. It will calm your mind and nervous system and help to relieve insomia. This pose is a seated version of Supported Relaxation Pose, which is done lying down.

How to Do It:

1. Sit straight on a chair with your feet flat on the floor. Your neck and head should be aligned with your spinal column. Close your eyes and rest your hands in your lap. Breathe through your nose, peaceful and relaxed.

2. Relax each part of your body. Begin by focusing your attention to your feet and toes. Inhale and suggest to your feet and toes that they relax. Exhale and feel your feet and toes relaxing. Repeat this relaxation procedure with each individual body part.

3. Practice Yoga Observation Meditation.

4. Relax all efforts and rest in the stillness for as long as you wish.

DOWNWARD-FACING DOG WITH CHAIR
(MODIFIED ADHO MUKHA SVANASANA)

What It Does: It stretches and strengthens the entire body, including the back muscles and hamstrings, and relieves stiffness in the neck and shoulders. As an inversion pose, Downward-Facing Dog also im-

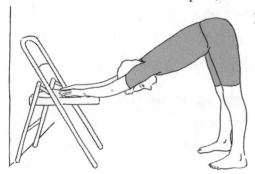

proves circulation to the head and upper body. Using the chair will help you maintain proper alignment in this pose, especially if you are stiff or weak. Be sure to place the chair against a wall to keep it from slipping. As you grow stronger and more flexible, follow this pose with Upward-Facing Dog with Chair, which follows, and try doing Downward-Facing Dog on the floor (see page 77).

How to Do It:

1. Place your hands on the front edge of the chair seat and step back until your arms are straight and your feet are slightly behind your hips, hip-width apart. If you're very stiff and the chair seat is too low for you to rest your arms on it comfortably, turn the chair around and practice with your hands resting on the chair back.

2. Stretch your spine and shoulders by pushing against the chair, stretching your fingertips forward and your buttocks back. Press your heels to the floor. Be in the moment and breathe!

3. Come out of the pose by bending your knees and taking a step forward with the right foot. Then step forward with the left and straighten to standing. Sit down in the chair if you need to rest, or progress to Upward-Facing Dog with Chair.

UPWARD-FACING DOG WITH CHAIR
(MODIFIED URDHVA MUKHA SVANASANA)

What It Does: It stretches and strengthens the entire body, especially the arms and shoulders. Using the chair will help you maintain proper alignment in this pose, especially if you are stiff or weak. Be sure to place the chair against a wall to keep it from slipping. As you grow stronger, do this pose directly after doing Downward-Facing Dog with Chair.

How to Do It:

1. Begin in Downward-Facing Dog with Chair position. Grip the sides of the chair seat and step back until your arms are straight and your feet are slightly behind your hips and are hip-width apart.

2. Press down into the seat and shift your weight forward into your arms while raising your heels off the floor. Straighten your arms, pull your shoulders down, away from your ears, and press your

shoulder blades toward the floor. Open your chest and lift your sternum. Be in the moment and breathe!

3. Come out of the pose by lowering your heels to the floor, bending your knees, and taking a step forward with the right foot. Then step forward with the left foot and straighten to standing. Sit down in the chair if you need to rest.

MODIFIED TREE POSE *(MODIFIED VRKSASANA)*

What It Does: It improves balance, strengthens the legs, and increases the flexibility of the hips and groin. A belt or strap will help keep your foot from slipping and maintain your hip's open position. As you grow stronger and more balanced and confident, practice without the belt.

How to Do It:

1. Bend your right leg and wrap a belt or strap around your right ankle and thigh, holding the end of the belt with your right hand. With your left hand,

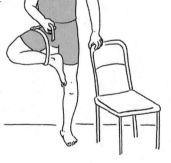

hold on to a chair or wall. Place the sole of your right foot at the top of your left inner thigh, bringing the foot as high up the leg as possible. Press the right knee back, trying to bring it in line with your right hip.

2. Gaze at a spot on the floor, but keep your eyes soft. Breathe gently.

3. If you have your balance, raise your left hand a few inches off the chair. Hold the pose for 3 or 4 breaths. If you sway or wobble, don't give up. Simply lean on the chair or wall to regain your balance before trying again.

4. Bring your right foot down slowly, letting the belt slip off your leg (control the motion). Stand steady, with both feet firmly grounded.

5. Repeat on the other side.

MODIFIED WARRIOR III
(MODIFIED VIRABHADRASANA III)

What It Does: It improves balance and stamina, strengthens the legs, and tones the hips and abdominals.

How to Do It:

1. Stand with your legs close together in Mountain Pose, about 2 feet from the wall. Lean forward and place both hands on the wall shoulder-width apart and above shoulder height. Press your shoulder blades down as you push against the wall with your hands.

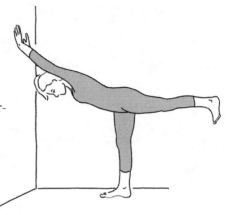

2. Exhale and slowly lift your left leg back. Straighten the left leg by actively pushing out through the heel. Keep the right leg straight and rooted to the ground. Gaze at a spot on the floor, but keep your eyes soft. Breathe gently.

3. Return to Mountain Pose. Repeat, raising the opposite leg. As you grow stronger and more confident and no longer need the wall to balance, give yourself enough room to extend both arms in front of you without touching the wall. Gaze at your outstretched hands.

EASY STOMACH LIFT *(MODIFIED UDDIYANA BANDHA)*

What It Does: It strengthens the stomach muscles to help support balancing poses and sustain good posture. Practice on an empty stomach. Be sure to place the chair against a wall to keep it from slipping.

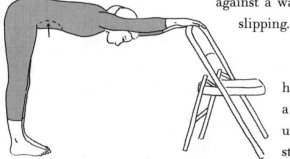

How to Do It:

1. Place your hands on the back of a chair and step back until your arms are straight and your feet are under your hips and are hip-width apart.

2. Press your hands into the chair and exhale forcefully out of your mouth. Close your mouth and bring your chin to your throat. Hold the exhalation and pull your abdomen back toward your spine and up toward your solar plexus.

3. Hold until you need to inhale; then relax the abdominals and inhale slowly.

4. Repeat.

MODIFIED DANCER POSE *(MODIFIED NATARAJASANA)*

What It Does: It stretches the quadriceps muscles, strengthens the standing leg, and improves balance. Practice while holding on to a wall or chair for additional support.

How to Do It:

1. Support yourself with your left hand resting on a chair back or wall. Bend your right knee and grasp your right ankle with your right hand.

2. Increase the stretch by pulling your right foot up behind you.

3. As you grow stronger and more balanced, slowly raise your left arm and look up at your fingers. Hold the pose for 10 seconds.

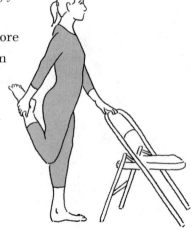

4. Repeat on the other side.

MODIFIED CHAIR POSE (MODIFIED UTKATASANA)

What It Does: It strengthens the lower body and improves balance.

How to Do It:

1. Stand in front of a chair with your feet hip-width apart. Inhale, bringing hands to a prayer position. Exhale, pull the abdomen in, and slowly squat until the backs of your thighs touch the chair.

2. Use the strength of your legs to rise slowly to standing.

3. Sit down in the chair if you need to rest.

4. As you build strength and confidence, squat without the chair.

chapter 4

Yoga Fountain of Youth

Researchers have found that regular exercise, yoga practice included, is an essential part of a long and healthy life. There is increasing evidence that many of the so-called age-related diseases, such as heart disease, hypertension, diabetes, cancer, and osteoporosis, as well as memory loss, are not linked inevitably to the aging process, but rather are the result of physical inactivity. While there is no magic pill to stop the effects of time, you can control your own destiny with these yoga postures and slow down most, if not all, of the declines associated with aging.

Longevity is the hot topic of the new millennium, as millions of baby boomers celebrate birthdays honoring their first fifty years. They're discovering that exercise isn't only about looking good, it's also the best—and safest—defense against the effects of aging in this era of long life spans. By the year 2030, one out of five people in the United States will be over age 65, and by 2050 nearly two billion people on the planet will be at least 60. Scientists believe that with exercise, medical advances, and healthier lifestyles, many of us will live to reach 100. Although we're still far from reaching the biblical patriarch Methuselah's 969, longer, healthier life spans are a modern-day reality.

Whatever your age, you should begin the Yoga Fountain of Youth Workout now to promote healthy aging. If you're in your twenties or thirties, aging probably isn't a major concern at the moment. But don't fool yourself. Bad habits, such as getting little or no exercise, sleeping too little, indulging in a fast-food diet, drinking to excess, or smoking, will take their toll on you, both internally and externally, in your middle years and beyond. This is the best time to achieve your optimal fitness and improve the quality of your life for today and for the decades to come. If you exercise regularly and intensely earlier in life, you won't have to work as hard to maintain your overall fitness level as you grow older. As early as your thirties, signs of aging do start to show up—from changes in metabolism, hormone levels, and lean body mass to decreases in aerobic capacity, strength, and flexibility. But don't despair! Yoga practice can slow and even reverse all of these declines at any age.

Move It or Lose It

When it comes to aging, there's truth to the saying "Move it or lose it." Some people have the misguided notion that at some point it's best to take it easy on an aging body—that is, to stop exercising. What a mistake! Although you may not be able to work out as intensely in your sixties as you did in your forties, yoga practice at any age can help you improve or maintain your fitness level and well-being.

If you can't find a 30-minute block of free time to exercise, or the thought of jogging makes your knees hurt, or you're bored by the treadmill, don't give up. This Yoga Fountain of Youth Workout incorporates the results of important recent studies that show that just three 10-minute intervals of moderate aerobic exercise a day can improve overall fitness. According to the recommendations of medical experts, 20 to 30 minutes of moderate activity over the course of a day, 3 times a week, will reward you with a long list of benefits.

Moderate physical activities include brisk walking, stair stepping, stationary cycling, and ashtanga vinyasa yoga. One of the misconceptions about yoga is that it doesn't provide a cardiovascular workout. However, a vigorous ashtanga vinyasa yoga practice, such as the Sun Salutation that follows, may be just as effective as many aerobic activities in promoting cardiovascular health, maintaining brain power, lowering the risk of cancer, strengthening bones and muscles, boosting immune system function, helping manage weight, and keeping skin looking young.

In ashtanga-style yoga we perform *vinyasas*, a continuous flow of poses. Ashtanga vinyasa features the same poses as hatha yoga, except that these poses are linked together in synchrony with the breath. Ashtanga vinyasa poses, such as those featured in Sun Salutation, are done one after another so that you're constantly moving between the poses. The result is a safe cardiovascular workout with the perfect blend of flexibility, strength, and aerobic conditioning.

Yoga for Heart Health

Dean Ornish, a clinical professor of medicine at the University of California, San Francisco, and founder of the Osher Center for Integrative Medicine, has proven scientifically that comprehensive life-style changes, including yoga practice, can reverse even severe coronary heart disease without drugs or surgery. The nonsurgical treatment and innovative program described in his best-selling book, *Dr. Dean Ornish's Program for Reversing Heart Disease* (Random House, 1990), includes hatha yoga, meditation, aerobic exercise, and a low-fat vegetarian diet. Dr. Ornish's program has proven so success-ful a defense against heart disease—the number one killer of both men and women in the United States—that some medical insurance companies now reimburse individuals who participate in it.

A plethora of health care providers, hospitals, and insurance companies confirm yoga's preventive benefits. Mehmet Oz, car-diac surgeon and author of *Healing from the Heart* (Dutton, 1998), is cofounder of the Complementary Care Center at New York–Presbyterian Hospital, which offers yoga, meditation, visualization, massage, and therapeutic touch. Dr. Oz encourages his cardiac pa-tients to engage in these mind-body therapies before and after heart bypass surgery, and the patients are often followed and studied through clinical trials. Major medical institutions around the coun-try have since opened their own complementary medicine programs that offer mind-body medicine, including yoga and meditation.

Various studies have shown that moderate physical activity, such as yoga Sun Salutation, strengthens the heart muscle and causes oxygen to be pumped through your circulatory system to your tissues more efficiently. The 1996 Surgeon General's Report on Physical Activity and Health concluded that, in addition to strengthening the heart, aerobic exercise benefits almost every organ and system in the body.

Yoga for Brain Health

Contrary to popular belief, memory loss is not a normal sign of aging. With the help of aerobic exercise, like the Sun Salutation, growing older doesn't have to mean a decline in your mental function. Dharma Singh Khalsa, author of *Brain Longevity* (Warner Books, 1997) and director of the Alzheimer's Prevention Foundation in Tucson, Arizona, recommends a brain longevity program that includes aerobic exercise, a healthful diet, and brain-boosting nutritional supplements to optimize mind power, improve memory, reduce the risk of Alzheimer's disease, and help prevent age-related memory loss. An important benefit of physical activity is that it increases circulation of blood to the brain, helping to maintain brain power and memory, and promoting attention and alertness. There is scientific evidence that those who exercise are the least likely to decline mentally.

Yoga Muscle Power

The Yoga Fountain of Youth Workout will also help strengthen and preserve muscle while improving balance and coordination. This becomes increasingly important as we age, since both men and women lose up to 30 percent of muscle mass between the ages of twenty and seventy. The faltering, shaky gait of the elderly is oftentimes caused by a loss of muscle and is a sign of myoatrophy, a treatable condition. Myoatrophy can be reversed with exercise that combines aerobic activities with weight-bearing exercises, such as those in the Yoga Fountain of Youth Workout.

The age-related loss of muscle also increases the risk of obesity as we grow older. Obesity, in turn, increases the possibility of contracting life-shortening diseases such as heart disease, diabetes, high blood pressure, and certain cancers. Since muscle burns more calories than fat, the more fit you are, the more calories your body burns while at rest. However, with aging, the metabolism (the rate at which your body burns calories) slows down as muscle mass dwindles, thereby making it easier to gain weight. To compensate for this metabolic slowdown we need to consume fewer calories and increase physical activity.

The Sun Salutation is the perfect mix of aerobic exercise and weight-bearing exercise. Yoga poses such as Downward-Facing Dog, Plank Pose, and Modified Plank Pose require you to support the weight of your body with your arms or legs as you move from one pose to another. The muscle-building benefits increase as you grow stronger and are able to hold the poses longer.

Go Upside Down

Throughout the millennia, yoga gurus and practitioners have promoted inversion poses—turning yourself upside down—to slow and even reverse the aging process. Tantra yoga tradition teaches that *amrita*, the nectar of immortality, resides at the seventh chakra within the cranium. Performing inversion postures such as the headstand stimulates the release of amrita, which drips down the body and is absorbed by the torso when you come out of the pose. This release of amrita is thought to promote perfect health and prevent aging.

Although there are no scientific studies that prove the existence of amrita, we do know that the pituitary and pineal glands, responsible for growth and sex hormones, are located in the center of the skull. It's possible that these pituitary and pineal glands may be stimulated to release their hormones when the body is inverted.

What is better understood is that turning the body upside down increases blood circulation to the upper body and to the brain. Yoga inversion postures, such as Supported Shoulderstand, Pose of Tranquility, Supported Plough, Dolphin, and Legs-up-the-Wall Pose, have multiple health benefits. The increased blood flow to the heart may reduce blood pressure by helping to reset the pressure-regulating reflexes. The lungs, throat, sinuses, and thyroid also benefit from improved circulation.

Many baby boomers are turning to antioxidant and Retin-A creams and cosmetic surgery to combat the visible signs of aging. However, a more natural and less expensive means to a youthful appearance and ageless, glowing skin are these inverted yoga poses, which increase circulation of blood to the skin's surface; the blood carries nutrients that slow skin-cell degeneration and collagen breakdown.

Before You Start

- If you're just beginning a fitness program, comfortably and gradually work up to the frequency and duration of exercise recommended in the following workout.
- Perform the vinyasas slowly, according to your own abilities. You should never be breathless or in pain. Pay attention to your body's signals of overexertion, such as pounding in your chest, dizziness, faintness, profuse sweating, or an inability to carry on a normal conversation. If any of these symptoms occur, you need to slow down! If the symptoms persist, see your doctor.
- Always consult your physician before beginning a new exercise program.

Your 4-Week Yoga Fountain of Youth Workout Plans

Select one of the following three Yoga Fountain of Youth Workout Plans for maximum longevity benefits. The vinyasas presented in this chapter include the Sun Salutation and inversion poses for Beginner, Intermediate, and Maintenance levels. You can begin the Yoga Fountain of Youth Workout after practicing the Basics and Easy Yoga Workout found in Chapters 2 and 3 for 2 weeks. Be aware that it may take you more than 2 weeks to do this routine comfortably, depending on your physical condition. If you feel comfortable and confident doing these poses, proceed to the Yoga Fountain of Youth Workout.

As you progress from Beginner to Maintenance over a period of months, you'll build your yoga practice up from 30 to 60 minutes a day, 3 to 5 days a week. For additional longevity benefits, you can incorporate the Yoga Back Workout, the 10-Minute Yoga Relief Workout, or the Yoga for Sexual Vitality Workout into your practice, as described in Chapters 5, 6, and 7.

While practicing the first vinyasa cycle, you may feel stiff and clumsy. By the second or third cycle, the movements will start flowing more easily and the rhythm of your breathing will come more naturally.

As you practice the vinyasas, focus not only on each pose, but also on the use of your breath. Breath links the postures together in vinyasa practice and energizes your aerobic exercise. During your

Yoga Fountain of Youth Workout, maintain deep, rhythmic breathing, synchronizing the flow of yoga postures with your inhalation and exhalation. A good rule of thumb is to inhale while bending backward and exhale during forward-bending postures. Ujjayi breathing is a classic pranayama (yoga breathing) technique often linked with vinyasa. During ujjayi breathing you keep your breath steady and controlled (see Chapter 2, "Before You Begin").

Vinyasa yoga's full-body workout and powerful combination of stretching with exercises for strength and balance will produce beneficial physical improvements within a short time. Your spine will become more supple and tight hamstrings will begin to release as you tone, firm, and strengthen your body.

Yoga Fountain of Youth Workout Plans

1. BEGINNER FOUNTAIN OF YOUTH WORKOUT

After practicing the Basics and Easy Yoga Workout found in Chapters 2 and 3 for 2 weeks, beginners should start with this workout. After you've finished this 4-week plan, you can proceed to the Intermediate Yoga Fountain of Youth Workout. Be aware that it may take you more than 4 weeks to do this routine comfortably, depending on your physical condition. Feel free to take as much time as you need before progressing to Intermediate practice.

For additional longevity benefits, you can incorporate the Yoga Back Workout, the 10-Minute Yoga Relief Workout, or the Yoga for Sexual Vitality Workout into your practice, as described in Chapters 5, 6, and 7.

Weeks 1 and 2

Workout Schedule: Practice Sun Salutation 3 days a week for 20 minutes, followed by 10 minutes of inversion poses and Cool Down.

Warm Up: Perform Sun Salutation once slowly, holding each posture for 5 breaths.

Sun Salutation: Perform 4 repetitions of Sun Salutation, holding each posture for 3 breaths.

Inversion Poses:

Legs-up-the-Wall Pose

Bridge Pose with Strap

Cool Down:

Supported Relaxation Pose

Weeks 3 and 4

Workout Schedule: Practice Sun Salutation 3 days a week for 30 minutes, followed by 10 minutes of inversion poses and Cool Down.

Warm Up: Perform Sun Salutation once slowly, holding each posture for 5 breaths

Sun Salutation: Perform 6 repetitions of Sun Salutation, holding each posture for 1 to 3 breaths.

Inversion Poses:

Supported Shoulderstand with Wall

Modified Fish Pose (page 168)

Cool Down:

Supported Relaxation Pose

2. INTERMEDIATE FOUNTAIN OF YOUTH WORKOUT

After practicing the Beginners workout, begin this Intermediate Yoga Fountain of Youth Workout. Be aware that it may take you more than 4 weeks to do this routine comfortably, depending on your physical condition. Feel free to take as much time as you need before progressing to Maintenance practice.

For additional longevity benefits, you can incorporate the Yoga

Back Workout, the 10-Minute Yoga Relief Workout, or the Yoga for Sexual Vitality Workout into your practice, as described in Chapters 5, 6, and 7.

Weeks 1 and 2

Workout Schedule: Practice Sun Salutation 4 days a week for 30 minutes, followed by 10 minutes of inversion poses and Cool Down.

Warm Up: Perform Sun Salutation once slowly, holding each posture for 5 breaths.

Sun Salutation: Perform 6 repetitions of Sun Salutation, holding each posture for 1 to 3 breaths.

Inversion Poses:

Pose of Tranquility

Modified Fish Pose

Cool Down:

Supported Relaxation Pose

Weeks 3 and 4

Workout Schedule: Practice Sun Salutation 5 days a week for 30 minutes, followed by 10 minutes of inversion poses and Cool Down.

Warm Up: Perform Sun Salutation once slowly, holding each posture for 5 breaths

Sun Salutation: Perform 6 repetitions of Sun Salutation, holding each posture for 1 to 3 breaths.

Inversion Poses:

Dolphin Headstand Preparation

Supported Plough Pose

Cool Down:

Supported Relaxation Pose

3. MAINTENANCE FOUNTAIN OF YOUTH WORKOUT

Congratulations! At this point, you've mastered the Beginner and Intermediate Fountain of Youth Workouts. I'm sure you're looking and feeling great. Do the Maintenance Fountain of Youth Workout to continue to build and maintain your longevity, strength, cardiovascular fitness, and flexibility benefits.

For additional longevity benefits, you can incorporate the Yoga Back Workout, the 10-Minute Yoga Relief Workout, or the Yoga for Sexual Vitality Workout into your practice, as described in Chapters 5, 6, and 7.

Weeks 1 and Beyond

Workout Schedule: Practice Sun Salutation 5 days a week for 30 minutes, followed by 10 minutes of inversion poses and Cool Down. If your schedule is busy, you can break up this routine. For example, you can practice Sun Salutation for 15 minutes in the morning with Cool Down and then do an additional 15 minutes in the evening with 10 minutes of inversion poses and then Cool Down.

Warm Up: Perform Sun Salutation once slowly, holding each posture for 5 breaths.

Sun Salutation: Perform 6 repetitions of Sun Salutation, holding each posture for 1 to 3 breaths.

Inversion Poses—Choose two from the following:

Legs-up-the-Wall Pose

Bridge Pose with Strap

Supported Shoulderstand with Wall

Pose of Tranquility

Dolphin Headstand Preparation

Supported Plough Pose

Plus:

Modified Fish Pose

Cool Down:

Supported Relaxation Pose

SUN SALUTATION
(SURYA NAMASKAR)

This ancient, classic yoga routine is traditionally done at sunrise, but can of course be practiced at any time of day, and is a complete workout for body and mind.

1. Mountain Pose (Tadasana): Stand with your feet together, legs straight, kneecaps tightened and pulled up, weight distributed evenly, and hands in prayer position over your heart center. Tilt your pelvis under, with your abdomen pulled in and shoulders relaxed and pulled down, away from your ears. Lift your sternum toward the ceiling.

2. Standing Backbend: Inhale and raise your arms in a V overhead. Tighten your buttock muscles firmly to protect your lower back, lift your chest toward the ceiling, and bend backward. Pause for 3 seconds.

3. Standing Forward Bend (*Uttanasana*): Exhale, extending your arms forward, and fold your torso forward from the hips, abdomen in. Bend your knees slightly. Relax your face, head, neck, and shoulders toward the floor and lower your chest to your thighs. Place your hands on the floor, fingers in line with your toes.

4. Left Lunge (*Anjaneyasana*): Inhale, bending both knees and keeping your palms flat beside your feet. Step your right foot back, bringing your right knee to the floor. Stretch your chin up toward the ceiling. Your left knee should be directly over your left ankle (i.e., perpendicular to the floor).

5. Plank Pose (*Chaturanga Dandasana*): Exhale, bringing your left leg back to join your right, and extend your arms, as you would to begin a push-up. Keep your body straight, legs and arms extended and head in line with spine. Pull your stomach in. Hold for 1 or 2 breaths.

6. Modified Plank Pose (*Modified Chaturanga Dandasana*): Exhale, bending and lowering knees, chest, and chin to the floor. Hips are up, abdomen is in. This pose is similar to a modified women's push-up. Keep your elbows close to your body. If this is too difficult, go from Plank Pose to placing the body flat, face down on the floor. Then go into a modified women's push-up position.

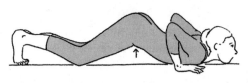

7. Cobra (*Bhujangasana*): Inhale, raising forehead, chin, and chest while arching your spine. Hips are on the floor. Elbows should be slightly bent and close to the body. Shoulders are pressed down and away from the ears. Tilt the pelvis under for lower-back protection. Pause for several breaths.

8. Downward-Facing Dog (*Adho Mukha Svanasana*): Exhale, lifting your hips up and back as you turn your body into an upside-down V. Keep your arms and legs straight and press your heels to the floor. Shoulders are pressed down, away from the ears.

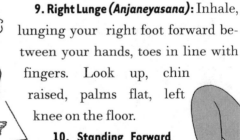

9. Right Lunge (*Anjaneyasana*): Inhale, lunging your right foot forward between your hands, toes in line with fingers. Look up, chin raised, palms flat, left knee on the floor.

10. Standing Forward Bend (*Uttanasana*): Exhale, pushing off with the toes of your left foot to bring the left foot forward to join the right. Upper body is folded forward from the hips, knees are slightly bent, hands are on either side of the feet.

11. Standing Backbend: Inhale, raising yourself upright and keeping your back straight, your arms extended overhead and knees slightly bent. Exhale and tighten your buttocks. Inhale, keeping your head between your arms; lift your sternum toward the ceiling and arch your spine backward. Pause for 3 seconds.

12. Mountain Pose *(Tadasana)*: Exhale; return to an upright position and bring your palms together. Take a few breaths, breathing in light and energy, exhaling tension and fatigue. Repeat Steps 2 through 12 on the opposite leg, bringing the left leg back for Step 4, then forward for Step 9, for a complete cycle.

Yoga Fountain of Youth Inversion Poses

LEGS-UP-THE WALL POSE (MODIFIED VIPARITA KARANI)

What It Does: This is a safe and simple way to get all the benefits of an inversion posture. It improves circulation to the upper body and the brain and calms the mind. When you grow stronger and more flexible and confident, practice Supported Shoulderstand with Wall and Pose of Tranquility.

How to Do It:

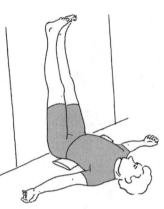

1. Sit on the floor beside the wall, with one shoulder as close to the wall as possible. Knees are bent.

2. Swing around and bring both legs up against the wall as you lie back on the floor. Extend your legs straight up the wall with your arms at your sides, keeping your buttocks against the wall. Breathing comfortably, stay in this position for 1 minute.

3. If your hamstring muscles are stiff and tight, bend your knees a bit. If your lower back, shoulders, and neck are uncomfortable, place a folded blanket or towel beneath them.

4. Come out of the pose by bending your knees, turning to one side, and slowly sitting up.

SUPPORTED SHOULDERSTAND WITH WALL
(SUPPORTED SARVANGASANA)

What It Does: This simpler, supported version of the full shoulderstand, known as the Queen of Asanas, will provide you with all of its antiaging benefits while toning and strengthening your entire body. Practice on a neatly folded blanket placed about 6 inches away from the wall. Always follow this posture with Fish Pose (see Modified Fish Pose, page 168).

How to Do It:

1. Sit on the folded blanket, with your side as close to the wall as possible and your knees bent.

2. Swing around and bring both legs up the wall, lying flat on your back with your shoulders on the blanket folds. Extend your legs straight up the wall, keeping your buttocks close to the wall.

3. Press the soles of your feet against the wall, bend your knees, and raise your buttocks off the floor, bringing yourself onto your shoulders. Bend your elbows and slide your hands up to your hips.

4. Open your chest by extending your elbows back, parallel to one another, toward the wall. Breathing comfortably, stay in this position for 30 to 60 seconds.

5. Come out of the pose by bringing your hips down the wall slowly and with control to the blanket, turning to the side, and sitting up.

POSE OF TRANQUILITY *(MODIFIED SALAMBA SARVANGASANA)*

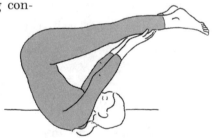

What It Does: Once you're feeling confident and strong doing Supported Shoulderstand with Wall, try this variation of Half Shoulderstand. To protect your neck, practice on a neatly folded towel or blanket, with your shoulders 3 to 4 inches from the folded edge and your head on the floor. Always follow with Fish Pose (see Modified Fish Pose, page 168).

How to Do It:

1. Lie on your back, feet together, hands at sides. Inhale and raise your legs straight up toward the ceiling.

2. Exhale and raise your hips off the floor, using your hands to push off. Support your pelvis with your hands cupped around your hips, your elbows close together. Keep your legs straight at a 45-degree angle.

3. Removing your elbows from the floor, place your hands on your thighs, knees, or lower legs, and balance on your shoulders.

4. Hold this balance for 30 to 60 seconds. Breathe comfortably.

5. To come out of the pose, bend both knees to your forehead and bring your hands to the floor. Slowly and with control, bring your hips to the floor. Straighten your legs and lower them to the floor. If your back and abdominals are weak, bend your knees to your forehead and lower your bent legs to the floor.

SUPPORTED PLOUGH POSE *(SUPPORTED HALASANA)*

What It Does: This simpler, supported version of Plough Pose bestows a long list of antiaging benefits. Full Plough should be practiced only with the supervision of an experienced teacher. Place your chair sideways approximately 8 to 12 inches from your head (see illustration). Do not proceed with this pose if you feel excessive pressure or pain in the back of the head or neck.

How to Do It:

1. Lie on your back, feet together, hands at sides. Inhale and raise your legs straight up toward the ceiling.

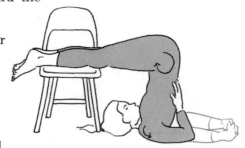

2. Exhale and raise your hips off the floor, using your hands to push off. Place your lower legs on the seat of the chair. Clasp your hands behind your torso and lengthen your arms away from your head. Pull your shoulders down, away from your ears, and rotate your shoulder blades toward your spine.

3. Rotate and press your pelvis under, elongating the spine. Now bend your arms at the elbows and place your hands on your back. Elbows are parallel and close together. Press the shoulders and elbows down as you elongate the spine.

4. Breathe comfortably in this position for 30 to 60 seconds.

5. To come out of the pose, bend both knees to your forehead and bring your hands to floor. Slowly and with control, bring your hips to the floor. Straighten your legs and lower them to the floor.

DOLPHIN HEADSTAND PREPARATION *(ARDHA SIRSANA)*

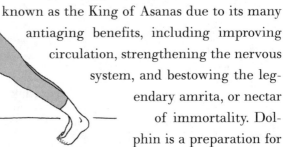

What It Does: This is a simpler, supported version of Headstand, known as the King of Asanas due to its many antiaging benefits, including improving circulation, strengthening the nervous system, and bestowing the legendary amrita, or nectar of immortality. Dolphin is a preparation for Headstand, which requires the supervision of a qualified instructor. Practice this on a mat with a neatly folded blanket or padding for your head.

How to Do It:

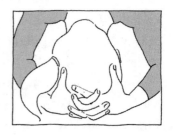

1. Kneel on the floor and then rest your forearms on the mat in front of you, so that your thighs and upper arms are perpendicular to the floor. Measure the distance between your elbows by placing your left fist against your right elbow. Elbows should be shoulder-width apart. Interlace

your fingers, forming a triangular base with your forearms. Place the crown of your head on the floor, supporting it with cupped hands.

2. Exhale and lift your hips, straightening your knees, with the balls of your feet pressing into the mat. Press your upper arms and the center of your forearms (the ulna) into the mat to create leverage. Draw your shoulders away from your neck. The top of each wrist is directly over the bottom of the wrist, not tilting in or out.

3. Inhale, push down on your forearms, and lift your head a few inches off the floor. Exhale and bring the crown of your head back down to the mat. Repeat 3 times.

4. Bend your knees and lower them to the floor. Keep your head down for a few moments before sitting up.

BRIDGE POSE WITH STRAP *(MODIFIED SETU BANDHASANA)*

What It Does: This beginner's backbend is an excellent complementary posture for inversions. Doing the Bridge Pose helps to stretch the abdominal muscles, opens the chest area, increases flexibility in the spine, and firms the buttocks. If you're stiff, place a strap around your ankles to assist in the alignment of your feet, ankles, knees, and hips.

How to Do It:

1. Lie on your back. Bend both knees and place your feet flat on the floor, hip-width apart. Place a strap around your ankles.

2. Tilt your pelvis, pressing the small of your back gently to the floor (see Pelvic Tilt, 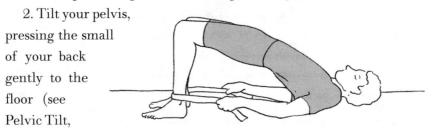 page 27). Inhale. Keep the back of your head on the floor. Slowly exhaling, raise your hips up to the middle of the shoulders one vertebra at a time, using your abdominals (building a bridge). Stabilize by pressing down on your heels and holding on to the strap. Tighten your buttocks and continue to tilt your pelvis under. Hold for 6 seconds.

3. Exhaling slowly, lower your spine to the floor, one vertebra at a time.

Yoga for a Youthful Back

I f you've always thought a stiff or painful back was an inevitable consequence of aging, the Yoga Back Workout in this chapter
will change your mind. Whether you're searching for a lasting fix
for nagging back pain or want to prevent future backaches, this
yoga routine is for you. By practicing these yoga postures, you can
enjoy a healthy, pain-free back and stay youthful and active for a lifetime.

Practicing yoga has been shown to be one of the most effective
and healthy ways to relieve back pain caused by weak or tight muscles, poor posture, overexertion, injury, a sedentary lifestyle, or tension. Many health professionals prescribe yoga to alleviate back
troubles. With regular practice, yoga can help prevent future back
problems by helping you build back strength, release tension, im-

prove structural alignment, and increase the tone and flexibility of your abdominals, hamstrings, and hips.

From a yoga point of view, overall wellness and longevity begin with a healthy spine. Over the millennia, yoga has evolved to promote the health of the spine by increasing the resiliency and strength of the back. The spine is also thought to be where the *kundalini* energy (the psychospiritual energy force) resides. In addition to the kundalini, yoga masters believe, there are over seventy-two thousand subtle energy channels, or *nadis,* in the body through which life force (prana) flows and connects to the body's energy centers, or *chakras,* all of which originate in the spine. Certain esoteric yoga practices concentrate on purifying the energy channels and raising the kundalini of the spine so that prana can flow easily, bringing perfect health along with an awakening to a higher consciousness.

Advanced age, a sedentary lifestyle, lack of exercise, injuries, poor posture, or inadequate nutrition can lead to decreased blood circulation to and through the spine. This, in turn, causes the discs of the spine to shrink, while the spaces between the vertebrae shorten. Over time the spine gradually stiffens and compresses, and you lose inches from your height. Your back may then hunch over and pinch the spinal nerves, further limiting circulation. A hunched back may also create problems with your breathing by compromising your lung capacity and further reducing the circulation to and nourishment of every cell in your body. This dreadful chain of events, which sets up the possibility of even more ailments and complications, unfortunately is an all-too-common consequence of the toxic, sedentary lifestyle so prevalent in our society.

It's a sobering scenario, but not an inevitable one if you take proper preventive measures. Doing yoga makes it possible to keep your spine youthful, supple, and strong. Living proof of yoga's effectiveness are the many practitioners who appear years younger and far healthier than their chronological, but inactive, peers.

Back Basics

Research studies show that at least eight out of ten adults will suffer from back pain sometime in their lives. For many of them the pain is chronic. Back pain is cited as the second most common reason people seek out a doctor (it's second only to the common cold). If you're fortunate enough to have a healthy back, take steps now to keep it that way. If you neglect the health of your back or you're unknowingly abusing it, you may be inviting future back injury.

By understanding how the spine works, you can act to heal your back pain and prevent future injuries. Your body is held upright by your spine's complex network of bony vertebrae that are padded by cartilage discs and surrounded by muscles and ligaments. These cartilage discs allow for flexibility in spinal movements and function as shock absorbers as we walk, run, and jump.

Despite the spine's remarkable structure, it can be susceptible to problems. Back pain most often appears in the lower back or the sacroiliac (SI) joint—where the sacrum and ilium meet in the pelvis. The SI joint is held together by strong yet pliable ligaments designed to maintain stability in the pelvis as we stand and walk. Lower-back pain is often the result of stress in the SI joint, caused by an accident, poor muscle tone, bad posture, or inappropriate, counterproductive movement patterns. All can strain the ligaments and alter stability in the lower back and pelvis, causing discomfort and painful flare-ups.

The best way to treat and prevent SI injury is to move the pelvis and spine together during yoga poses, such as Head-to-Knee pose. Backward-bending movements, as in Bridge Pose, will help strengthen and stabilize the SI joint and lower back.

Back pain may also be caused by damaged cartilage discs that have lost their shock-absorbing ability. An accident sustained in lifting a heavy weight improperly, or poor alignment and movement patterns, may cause the supporting spinal ligaments to weaken or tear. This causes the gel-like disc to bulge or herniate out, creating back pain. If the herniated disc presses on an adjacent spinal nerve, it can cause referred pain in the hip and leg.

Practicing gentle forward bends, such as the Seated Forward Bend in Chair and Modified Spread-Leg Forward Bend, trains you to bend forward properly without pain or strain to the cartilage discs and the SI joint. You'll no longer shy away from forward-bending movements, such as those made in shopping, stooping to pick up a child, or doing housework or gardening chores.

Scoliosis, or curvature of the spine, is another common cause of back pain. In scoliosis, the spine curves from side to side in an S shape, and this may result in one shoulder jutting higher than the other or a similar problem with the hip joints. Functional scoliosis can result from poor posture or unbalanced movement patterns. Structural scoliosis, which is more serious, can appear during adolescence. Its causes are not well understood.

Yoga poses strengthen the spinal muscles and promote spinal alignment and healthy posture and movement patterns. Gentle twists, such as Seated Twist, can improve spinal curvature, tone your spine, and relieve tension.

Tight hamstrings and abdominals—often the result of poor posture—are also culprits in creating back strain and pain. Hamstrings are the muscles in the back of your thighs, and chronically tight hamstrings can affect posture and compromise the health of your lower back. Tightness in the abdominal muscles occurs when there's an imbalance between abdominal and back muscles. This muscular imbalance can arise from the best intentions, such as a commitment to an abdominal strengthening routine of sit-ups and crunches. Combined with total neglect of the back muscles, this limited exercise routine can tighten the abdominals while the back muscles weaken and become overstretched.

Gentle hamstring stretches, such as Modified Reclining Big-Toe Pose, will lengthen the hamstrings without compromising your back. You can stretch and balance tight abdominals by doing Yoga Sit-Ups, Half Boat Pose, and Modified Revolved Abdomen Pose.

Poor postural habits that lead to tight or weak muscles can contribute to back pain. Good posture improves more than just aesthetics; it substantially reduces the risk of pain and injury, especially in your lower back. Yoga teaches beautiful posture and the basics of body alignment, with poses such as Cow's-Head Pose and Modified Locust Pose. Yoga poses and body-mind disciplines are powerful tools to improve posture and relieve and prevent back pain. These healing movement combinations can be found in Pelvic Tilt, One-Legged Wind-Relieving Pose, and Yoga Sit-Up.

Yoga Back Soothers

Yoga poses performed correctly and with awareness, as in the Longevity Back Sequence, can treat and prevent many back problems. Adding self-massage techniques, such as *do-in* and acupressure, is an effective way to alleviate and prevent back pain. As discussed in Chapter 1, *do-in* and acupressure can help to relieve and prevent tension and tightness, promote flexibility in muscles, and increase blood circulation. The spinal cord contains multiple nerves that branch out to every part of the body, with important acupressure points located along the spine. Combining self-massage with yoga stretches enhances the healing benefits of the poses.

As discussed in Chapter 1, I've incorporated aspects of the body-mind disciplines Ideokinesis and Pilates into the following workout to enhance the benefits of yoga practice. These approaches restore strength and energy, integrate mind and body, and reeducate the body with respect to movement patterns to heal our bodies and allow us to carry out our activities more efficiently.

Before You Start

Improperly performed stretching, in doing yoga poses as well as in other activities, can also cause back pain and strain; it can aggravate scoliosis or even damage the SI joint or the spinal discs. For example, yoga poses that move the pelvis and sacrum in opposite directions, such as yoga twists, when done incorrectly can cause instability in the SI joint. Improperly performed yoga forward bends can also be especially risky for people with tight hamstrings or back problems. That is why the utmost attention should be paid to doing the poses correctly.

Keep in mind that, depending on the nature and severity of your back problem, yoga poses may not be helpful. If you have a history of lower-back pain, disc damage, or a recent lower-back injury, it may not be safe to do yoga. These poses should not be performed during the acute phase of any injury, including a back injury. Stop any exercise if your pain gets worse. Be sure to have a health care professional diagnose your back problem, and check with her or him before doing the following workout.

Yoga Back Workout

If your time is limited, the Yoga Back Workout can be practiced on its own. You will reap benefits even if you have only 15 minutes to do this yoga practice. For maximum longevity benefits, combine this workout with any of the Yoga Fountain of Youth Workouts in Chapter 4. For example, see the combination of the Maintenance Fountain of Youth Workout and the Yoga Back Workout that follows.

Be aware that it may take you more than 4 weeks to do this routine comfortably, depending on your physical condition. If you feel comfortable and confident doing the poses in Weeks 1 and 2, proceed to Weeks 3 and 4. Otherwise, stay with Weeks 1 and 2 until you feel strong enough to continue.

Weeks 1 and 2

Practice Schedule: Practice for 15 to 20 minutes, 3 days a week.

Yoga Back: For each workout, perform the seven poses of the Longevity Back Sequence, then choose at least one additional back pose.

Longevity Back Sequence: Do all seven poses.

Choose at Least One:

Seated Forward Bend in Chair

Seated Twist

Cow's-Head Pose

Modified Revolved Abdomen Pose

Weeks 3 and 4

Practice Schedule: Practice for 15 to 20 minutes, 3 days a week.

Yoga Back: For each workout, perform the seven poses of the Longevity Back Sequence, then choose at least one additional back pose.

Longevity Back Sequence: Do all seven poses.

Choose at Least One:

Half Boat Pose

Bridge Pose

Modified Head-to-Knee Pose

Modified Locust Pose

Modified Spread-Leg Forward Bend

Maintenance Fountain of Youth and Yoga Back Workout

A combination of the Yoga Back Workout and the Maintenance Fountain of Youth Workout will help you to strengthen your back, prevent and relieve back problems, and build and maintain your cardiovacular fitness, strength, and flexibility.

Week 1 and Beyond

Workout Schedule: Practice Sun Salutation 5 days a week for 30 minutes, followed by two inversion poses, plus Modified Fish Pose (see page 168) and Cool Down. On practice days 1, 3, and 5, follow with Yoga Back Workout poses. Finish with Cool Down.

Warm Up: Perform Sun Salutation once slowly, holding each posture for 5 breaths.

Sun Salutation: Perform 6 repetitions of Sun Salutation, holding each posture for 1 to 3 breaths.

Inversion Poses—Choose two from the following:

Legs-up-the-Wall Pose

Bridge Pose with Strap

Supported Shoulderstand with Wall

Pose of Tranquility

Dolphin Headstand Preparation

Supported Plough Pose

Plus:

Modified Fish Pose

Yoga Back Poses: On practice days 1, 3, and 5, do 15 to 20 minutes of Yoga Back Workout.

Cool Down: Supported Relaxation Pose

The Longevity Back Sequence

This simple, 10-minute routine can treat and prevent many back problems and keep your spine youthful, supple, and strong. The following seven yoga poses should be practiced one after the other.

1. PELVIC TILT IN CONSTRUCTIVE REST POSITION (MODIFIED SAVASANA)

What It Does: In Ideokinesis, the bent-knee Modified Relaxation Pose (Modified Savasana) is called the

Constructive Rest position. In this position, gravity naturally releases your muscles, thereby allowing you the opportunity to do mental imagery work. The Pelvic Tilt press, hold, and release action massages tension and stress out of the lower back while bringing fresh, oxygenated blood into the muscles and tissues. It is essential to tighten the buttock muscles firmly to protect and stabilize your lower back and activate the abdominals. To relieve any discomfort in the neck and throat, place a folded blanket underneath your head.

How to Do It:

1. Lie on your back, bending your knees so that your feet are flat on the mat, hip-width apart. Rest your hands on your abdomen or place your arms out to the sides as in Supported Relaxation Pose (see page 31). Relax your shoulders and pull them down, away from your ears. Align your neck and head with your spine. Close your eyes.

2. Allow the weight of your bones to sink toward the floor. Mentally scan your entire body, especially your spine and your lower back, noting any muscular contractions. Now surrender your muscles to the pull of gravity, and sink further into the floor.

3. Inhale and allow your lower back to arch naturally. Exhale, tightening the buttock muscles, tilting the pelvis under, and pulling

the abdomen in. Press the small of your back gently to the mat. Hold for 5 seconds, then relax all efforts. Move into the next pose.

2. ONE-LEGGED WIND-RELEASING POSE
(ARDHHA PAVANAMUKTASANA)

What It Does: This pose relieves sciatica and lower-back pain, ache, or stiffness. It also stretches the lower-back muscles.

How to Do It:

1. From Constructive Rest position, bring your right knee in to your chest. Comfortably hug your right 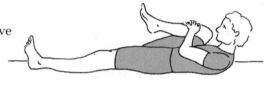 thigh to your chest. If your shoulders are tight, you can loop a strap or belt around the front of your right knee.

2. Slowly straighten your left leg with left foot flexed, making sure that your pelvis and right buttock remain on the floor and are aligned with your torso. If your pelvis comes off the floor or you feel pain, keep the left leg bent.

3. Release any muscular tension you may have on the front of the

left hip socket, surrendering your muscles to the pull of gravity as you sink into the floor.

4. Inhale as you hug your right knee gently toward your body and contract the muscles of your left leg and flexed foot. As you grow stronger and more confident and pain-free, bring your nose forward to your right knee. Keep your shoulders down, away from your ears. Hold for 5 seconds. Exhale and release.

5. Smoothly breathe in and out. Repeat on the left side. Repeat on each side.

3. KNEES-TO-CHEST POSE (PAVANAMUKTASANA)

What It Does: It relieves sciatica and lower-back pain, ache, or stiffness, and it stretches the lower-back muscles.

How to Do It:

1. From Constructive Rest position, bring your knees in to your chest. Hold the back of your thighs and bring the thighs as close to your rib cage as possible.

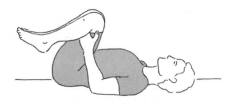

2. Inhale. Exhale and slowly pull the thighs toward the chest, lifting your buttocks slightly off the floor.

3. Inhale and release your buttocks back down to the floor. Breathe and hold the pose for 30 to 60 seconds.

4. YOGA SIT-UP

What It Does: This pose is enhanced by the addition of Pilates abdominal strengthening principles. The Yoga Sit-Up utilizes the Pelvic Tilt while contracting the abdominals, thereby protecting and 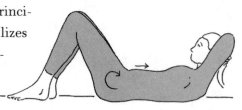 strengthening the lower back while fully engaging the abdominal muscles.

How to Do It:

1. From Constructive Rest position, place your hands behind the base of your head. Keep your elbows out to the sides.

2. Inhale, then exhale, tilting your pelvis under and pulling your abdomen in.

3. Inhale, then exhale, lifting your head and shoulders off the

floor as far as comfortably possible while keeping your neck relaxed and your pelvis tilted under. Exhale and hold, deepening the contraction of the abdominals.

4. Inhale and return to the starting position.

5. Repeat up to 10 times.

5. MODIFIED RECLINING BIG TOE POSE
(MODIFIED SUPTA PADANGUSTHASANA)

What It Does: It increases the flexibility and strength of the hamstrings and legs, and it helps release tightness in the back.

How to Do It:

1. In Constructive Rest position, wrap a belt or strap around the ball of your right foot.

2. Inhale and straighten your right leg toward the ceiling. Exhale, tilting the pelvis under. If you're unable to fully straighten the right leg, keep it bent, so that your sit bones (the bones you can feel in your buttocks) drop toward the floor.

2. Inhale and bend the right leg. Exhale and straighten the right leg again, to the point where you are stretching comfortably but any further stretching would cause discomfort. Draw the right leg closer to your face, applying gentle leverage with the belt. Work up to holding for 2 or 3 breaths.

4. As you grow more flexible, keep your right leg straight and actively straighten your left leg, pressing the back of the leg into the floor. Actively push out through the heels of both feet. Return the right leg to the floor.

5. Repeat on the other side. Once you've established this basic pose, practice without the belt, placing both hands around your thigh, calf, or ankle.

6. CAT-COW WITH ACUPRESSURE
(CHAKRAVAKASANA VARIATION)

What It Does: This posture flow stretches the lower back, lengthens and strengthens the spinal muscles, increases circulation to the spinal discs, and helps relieve back tension and pain. It stimulates spinal acupressure points along the lower back, called the Gates of Life, which regulate the central nervous system.

How to Do It:

1. Get down on all fours, with your hands directly below your shoulders and your knees below your hips. Your back should be straight and your palms flat on the floor, your torso like a tabletop.

2. Inhaling, lift your head and drop your abdomen, arching your lower back.

3. In a flowing motion, return to table position as you exhale, then round your back like a cat. Pull your stomach up toward your spine while looking down at the floor. Hold. Release, relaxing spine and abdomen.

4. Establish a smooth flow of inhaling, lower back arched, and exhaling, back rounded. Repeat 10 times.

7. MODIFIED CHILD'S POSE WITH SELF-MASSAGE (MODIFIED SALAMBA BALASANA)

What It Does: Modified Child's Pose provides deep relaxation and stretching of the back muscles. It relieves back tension, pain, and fatigue. The addition of the self-massage technique *do-in* to this pose enhances the healing benefits to the back.

How to Do It:

1. Kneel in front of a bolster or folded blankets. Knees are wide apart, big toes are touching. Put the bolster between your thighs, drawn up to the groin. If sitting on your ankles is uncomfortable, place a pillow under your ankles and feet.

2. Inhale. Then exhale slowly and bend forward, lowering your torso to rest on the bolster. Relax your arms around the support. Turn your face to one side. Relax deeply. Breathe comfortably.

3. With lightly closed fists, gently tap your lower back and pelvis several times.

4. Now relax all efforts. Inhale healing breath into your back. As you exhale, relax your back, visualizing it elongating while releasing all tension and pain. Continue your visualization as you breathe comfortably.

5. Rest for as long as you wish. Return to kneeling slowly.

Additional Yoga Back Poses

SEATED FORWARD BEND IN CHAIR *(MODIFIED UTTANASANA)*

What It Does: It stretches the back and helps prevent lower-back strain. As you grow stronger and more flexible, practice Modified Spread-Leg Forward Bend.

How to Do It:

1. Sit straight on a chair with your legs together and feet flat on the floor.

2. Inhale. Exhale, rounding your shoulders and spine forward, one vertebra at a time. Lower your forehead to your knees, laying chest on thighs as your arms hang down by your legs. Feel your back and shoulder muscles stretch as you relax in the position for 3 breaths.

3. Place your hands on your knees and slowly roll up, one vertebra at a time, raising your head last. Repeat.

SEATED TWIST
(MODIFIED BHARADVAJASANA)

What It Does: It increases spine and neck flexibility, and it releases tension and fatigue from the back muscles. This is especially helpful for individuals suffering from scoliosis, as it can help remedy spinal curvature.

How to Do It:

1. Sit straight on a chair with your legs together and feet flat on the floor. Inhale, lengthen your spine, and place your left hand on your right knee and your right hand on the back of the chair.

2. Exhale and gently twist your body to the right, turning your belly, then your chest, then your shoulders, then your head, directing your gaze over your right shoulder. Keep your shoulder blades down and in. Hold for 3 breaths.

3. Slowly return to center, beginning with the belly, then the chest, shoulder, head, and eyes.

4. Repeat the twist to the left.

MODIFIED HEAD-TO-KNEE POSE
(MODIFIED JANU SIRSASANA)

What It Does: It increases the flexibility and strength of the spine, hips, and legs and tones the abdomen and abdominal organs. As you grow more flexible, dispense with the belt and the blanket.

How to Do It:

1. Sit on the floor, with a folded blanket under your hips and your legs extended in front of you. Bend your right leg and rest the sole of your right foot on your left groin. Wrap a belt or strap around the ball of your left foot.

2. Inhale and lengthen your torso, pulling up from the waist, letting your sternum rise. Press your shoulder blades down.

3. Exhale and fold forward, leading with the sternum and rotating to the left in order to center your torso over your straight left leg. Allow your pelvis to rotate forward with the spine in a straight line.

Don't curve the upper back as you reach forward. Performing these actions properly will help prevent SI joint injury. If you feel pain or discomfort in your back or leg, bend your left leg as much as necessary to alleviate it. Never force yourself.

4. Inhale and elongate the spine, lengthening your torso forward. Exhale and stretch to your edge, the point beyond which you would feel discomfort. Work up to holding for 2 or 3 breaths.

5. Inhale and come up slowly. Repeat on the other side.

MODIFIED REVOLVED ABDOMEN POSE
(MODIFIED JATHARA PARIVARTANASANA)

What It Does: It exercises the external and internal oblique muscles and strengthens the abdominal wall. It also stretches the rotator muscles of the outer hips, and this enhances the proper functioning of the sacroiliac joint.

How to Do It:

1. Lie on your back, knees pulled in toward your chest. Keep your lower back in contact with the floor. Straighten your arms out to the sides in a T position at shoulder level, palms down.

2. Exhale. Keeping your knees together, slowly lower them to the

right while keeping your shoulders in contact with the floor. Touch the floor with the outside of your right foot. Gaze toward your left hand.

3. Relax for 3 full breaths.

4. Inhale; then use your abdominal muscles and raise your knees back to starting position.

5. Repeat on the left side.

6. Repeat for 2 more cycles.

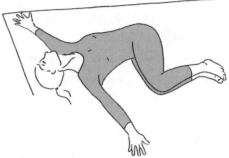

HALF BOAT POSE
(MODIFIED NAVASANA)

What It Does: It tones and strengthens your abdominal muscles, bringing them into balance with your back muscles.

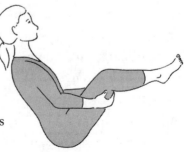

How to Do It:

1. Sit on the floor with your knees bent, feet flat on the floor hip-

width apart. With your hands, hold the backs of your thighs, close to your knees.

2. Lean back, lifting your legs so your calves are parallel to the floor. Balance on your sit bones.

3. Inhale, then exhale. Now straighten your arms forward, parallel to the floor, palms facing each other. If this is too difficult, hold the backs of your thighs with your hands. Draw your navel back toward your spine. Work up to holding this pose for 30 seconds. Balance and breathe!

4. Exhale and bring your feet to the floor.

5. Repeat 3 times.

BRIDGE POSE *(SETU BANDHASANA)*

What It Does: This is a complementary pose to develop a perfect balance of abdominal and back strength and suppleness. It strengthens and stabilizes the sacroiliac joint and lower back.

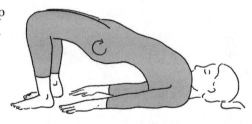

How to Do It:

1. Lie on your back, arms along your sides, your palms down. Bend both knees and place your feet flat on the floor, hip-width apart.

2. Tilt your pelvis, pressing the small of your back gently to the floor. Inhale. Now slowly exhale as you raise your hips, then your back, one vertebra at a time, to the middle of the shoulders (building a bridge). Stabilize by pressing down on your heels. Tighten your buttocks and tilt your pelvis under. Hold for 6 seconds.

3. Exhaling slowly, lower your spine to the floor, one vertebra at a time.

COW'S-HEAD POSE *(GOMUKHASANA)*

What It Does: It improves posture by developing flexibility in the chest, shoulders, upper back, hips, and legs. It helps to correct rounded shoulders.

How to Do It:

1. Begin seated, with legs extended in front of you. Cross your bent right knee over your left leg so that your right foot rests beside your left hip. Rocking back on your sit bones, bend your left leg so that your left foot rests beside your right hip. Now raise your right

arm overhead and reach behind you as if to scratch your back. Reach your left arm behind your back, hand pointing up. Clasp your hands firmly between your shoulder blades. (If you can't clasp hands, hold one end of a towel or strap with your left hand and grab the other end with your right hand. Gradually work your hands closer together on the towel.)

2. Keep your head erect, feel the stretch, and hold the pose for 3 slow, deep breaths.

3. Unclasp your hands, straighten your legs, and repeat on the other side.

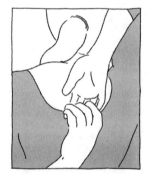

MODIFIED LOCUST POSE
(MODIFIED SALABHASANA)

What It Does: It strengthens the back—especially the erector spinae muscles—and the leg hamstrings. It improves posture by reducing rounding of the upper back. Doing this pose will also help individu-

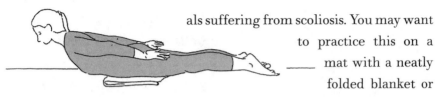

als suffering from scoliosis. You may want to practice this on a _____ mat with a neatly folded blanket or some padding underneath your chest, abdomen, and hips.

How to Do It:

1. Lie face down on the mat with your arms stretched down along your sides, your palms turned up, and your forehead on the floor.

2. Inhale, raise your arms upward, and lift your chest, keeping your gaze toward the floor. Reach your hands toward your toes. To protect your lower back, pull your abdomen in and tuck your pelvis under; tighten your buttocks and keep both hips firmly on the mat. Hold for 3 seconds.

3. Exhale, lowering your chest and arms to the mat.

4. Repeat the entire exercise twice.

MODIFIED SPREAD-LEG FORWARD BEND
(MODIFIED PRASARITA PADA UTTANASANA)

What It Does: Performed with a block, this will help release and stretch tight hips; hamstrings, and abdominals as well as prevent lower-back strain. Use an appropriately sized block or similar prop that suits your flexibility needs or limitations. As you grow stronger and more flexible, replace the block with a book, until you can comfortably reach the floor with your hands.

How to Do It:

1. Place the block about 1 foot in front of you between your wide-spread legs (your feet should be 3 to 4 feet apart).

2. Inhale, then exhale, folding forward from the hips and placing your hands on the block. Pull your abdomen in.

3. Hang comfortably for 6 to 8 breaths.

4. Come to standing, pulling your abdominals in.

chapter 6

Yoga to Relieve Aches and Pains

No More Pain

At one time or another, most of us have suffered from aches and pains in our joints or some other part of our body. Right now, you may be one of the millions of people who suffer from arthritis, knee problems, repetitive strain injury, or some other musculoskeletal problem. Well, say good-bye to your aches and pains! The soothing workout that follows will help to ease the pain you feel now and prevent future pain naturally by relaxing your body, relieving stress, and gently stretching your muscles. These simple yoga postures will keep your joints and muscles supple, helping you to move more easily. Practicing yoga has been shown to be one of the most effective ways to restore joint health, relieve muscular tension, and improve strength.

Many think of arthritis as a disease of the aged, but according to the Centers for Disease Control and Prevention (CDC) in Atlanta, arthritis affects people of all ages, and is the leading cause of disability among Americans, both young and old. Over forty-three million Americans have arthritis, and that number is expected to increase as baby boomers move through middle age and life expectancies increase. Researchers predict that by the year 2020 the number of people with arthritis will increase by 57 percent to over sixty million people. That's a whopping one in five Americans. For women, the incidence is expected to climb even higher—to one in four.

The ubiquitous ache of arthritis makes it one of the world's most common medical complaints. It's no surprise, then, that health experts warn that arthritis will become a major public health problem unless we actively embrace positive lifestyle interventions.

One of the interventions recommended by the CDC is low-impact exercise, such as the yoga practice presented here. Studies have shown that exercise is vital in preventing arthritis. Exercising helps to strengthen the muscles, and this, in turn, stabilizes the joints, maintains proper body alignment, and reduces the risk of injury. Yoga teaches the basics of good posture, moving painful and deformed joints back toward their normal position.

Yoga also helps reduce pain by providing a therapeutic combination of exercise, stress relief, breathing, and relaxation. This yoga program prevents the fight-or-flight response created by chronic stress and pain, which can begin a vicious circle of muscle tension, constricted blood circulation, and shallow chest breathing. Yoga's gentle stretches help reduce painful tension and muscle spasms and increase circulation. This special type of yoga practice will increase your blood flow, helping you to remove built-up toxins from your painful joints and muscles. Yoga in and of itself is not a cure-all for any specific condition, but it can be used as a complementary therapy to combat arthritis.

Another arthritis intervention recommended by the CDC is preventing and reducing obesity. Being overweight is a major risk factor for contracting arthritis. When you think about it, it makes perfect sense. Extra weight is a burden your joints have to bear. Yoga exercise will help to keep off those unwanted and unhealthy pounds.

By practicing yoga you will help yourself to stay fit and active, thereby keeping your weight down and your joints pain-free.

Yoga to the Rescue

"Arthritis" is a broad term encompassing a group of more than one hundred diseases that cause pain and stiffness of joints, muscles, tendons, or internal organs. The two most prevalent forms of arthritis are osteoarthritis (OA), sometimes called wear-and-tear arthritis, which develops over time; and rheumatoid arthritis (RA), an autoimmune disease in which the immune system mistakenly attacks the joints. OA and RA are actually very different from one another, and require different treatment.

Osteoarthritis, by far the most common arthritic condition, is the result of gradual deterioration of cartilage (the smooth, lubricated cushioning between bones) in the weight-bearing joints, including those in the hips, spine, knees, hands, and wrists. As cartilage wears down and deteriorates it becomes rough and pitted, leaving parts of the exposed bones to grind together. This increases friction and results in stiffness, pain, joint deformity, and a decreased range of motion.

A variety of factors can contribute to the development of OA joint deterioration, including excess weight, the chronic wear and tear of daily activities, sports injuries or accidents, and jobs that involve repetitive stress. Computer users, professional athletes, and dancers are prone to such problems. Yoga poses such as Yoga Hip Rock, Bound Angle Pose, and Modified Warrior I gently and gradually ease the limitations in the lower body and hip joints and ultimately restore a greater range of motion.

OA frequently affects the knees, since they are among the most often injured and abused joints in the body. The knee is a shallow, unstable joint, and its ligaments are especially vulnerable to twisting or side-bending forces. The yoga poses described in this chapter help to prevent injuries by stretching and strengthening the muscles around the knee joints and promoting proper leg and body alignment. Staff Pose and Warrior II Pose strengthen the quadriceps muscles in the front of the thighs, help stabilize the knees, and keep the leg bones in proper alignment. Salute to Gods and Goddesses and Hero Pose stretch the quadriceps muscles and the feet. Half Lotus Pose, a classic meditation posture, teaches proper leg, ankle, and foot alignment and restores flexibility to the hips and legs. Stretches for the hamstrings (in the back of the thighs), such as Side Angle Variation, help stabilize the knees, and correct poor leg alignment and muscular imbalances.

A small but promising study of patients with OA of the hands, published in *The Journal of Rheumatology,* showed that yoga exercise resulted in reduced pain and increased grip strength and range of motion.

Another study, published in *The Journal of the American Medical Association*, suggests that yoga can be used to treat carpal tunnel syndrome (CTS), also known as repetitive strain injury (RSI). CTS, or nerve compression in the wrists, is a problem for people who perform continual, repetitive movements with their fingers, hands, and wrists. Needless to say, this condition is a near epidemic among computer users. CTS or RSI can cause chronic, debilitating pain in the hands, arms, neck, or upper back.

The researchers found that yoga practice eased the compression of the affected nerves, improved blood flow, created proper joint and muscle alignment, assisted healing, and helped to prevent both RSI and OA. They designed a yoga program to strengthen and stretch the joints and muscles in the upper body, including the shoulders, arms, and wrists.

For people suffering from hand and wrist OA and RSI, weight-bearing yoga poses must be modified to safely stretch and strengthen without stressing the upper body (see the chair yoga poses in Chapter 3). In addition, Eagle Pose safely stretches and strengthens the shoulders and arms, while the Namaste Hand Mudra gently stretches the wrists, hands, and fingers. With regular practice, wrist and hand strength should gradually increase.

Adding self-massage to yoga stretches enhances their healing benefits for OA, RA, and RSI. The Yoga Wrist Stretch can help ease strain from repetitive wrist movements, and the Yoga Finger Stretch increases circulation and flexibility in the fingers.

In rheumatoid arthritis, the immune system mistakenly attacks the joints as if they were foreign invaders, causing painful inflammation, severe pain, and physical deformity. The inflammation damages the joints, including the cartilage, and in severe cases may cause joint fusion. The joints of the feet, ankles, and hands are often affected, as well as the shoulders and hips. A regular, less vigorous exercise regimen, such as the Easy Yoga poses (see Chapter 3), can help relieve the effects of RA. In addition, Yoga Foot Stretch safely stretches the feet and ankles, and Prana Breathing helps you relax, relieve tension, and reenergize.

Guidelines for Yoga to Relieve Aches and Pains

Each of us must be aware of his or her own abilities and limitations. Be sure to observe the following guidelines in your yoga practice to help relieve aches and pains.

- Before you begin this yoga program, consult a physician about your arthritis.
- Begin this yoga program gradually. Don't rush or push yourself past your limits. Instead, work gently and steadily to increase your body's capabilities.
- Yoga poses should not be performed when a joint is inflamed, swollen, hot, or injured.
- Listen to your body and know the difference between healthy soreness and pain. Stop any exercise if you feel pain.
- You may want to warm up before yoga practice by taking a hot shower or bath, and stay warm by doing your yoga poses in a well-heated room. Alternatively, you can dress in warm clothing.
- Gradually work into a yoga pose. Don't hold the pose for an extended period of time. Instead, try several brief repetitions of each pose.

10-Minute Yoga Relief Workout

If your time is limited, the 10-Minute Yoga Relief Workout can be practiced on its own. You will reap benefits even if you have only 10 minutes to do this yoga practice. For maximum longevity benefits, combine this workout with any of the Yoga Fountain of Youth Workouts in Chapter 4. For example, see the combination of the Maintenance Fountain of Youth Workout and the 10-Minute Yoga Relief Workout that follows.

Be aware that it may take you more than 4 weeks to do this routine comfortably, depending on your physical condition. If you feel comfortable and confident doing the poses in Weeks 1 and 2, proceed to Weeks 3 and 4. Otherwise, stay with Weeks 1 and 2 until you feel strong enough to continue.

Weeks 1 and 2

Practice Schedule: Practice for 10 minutes, 3 days a week.

Yoga Relief Poses—Choose at least three from the following:

Yoga Finger Stretch

Yoga Wrist Stretch

Staff Pose

Yoga Hip Rock

Bound Angle Pose

Modified Warrior I

Prana Breathing

Weeks 3 and 4

Practice Schedule: Practice for 10 minutes, 3 days a week.

Poses to Relieve Aches and Pains—Choose at least three from the following:

Namaste Hand Mudra

Yoga Foot Stretch

Salute to Gods and Goddesses

Side Angle Variation

Warrior II

Hero Pose

Eagle Pose

Half Lotus

Maintenance Fountain of Youth and Yoga Relief Workout

A combination of the 10-Minute Yoga Relief Workout and the Maintenance Fountain of Youth Workout will help ease aches and pains and prevent future pain, as well as build and maintain your cardiovacular fitness, strength, and flexibility.

Week 1 and Beyond

Workout Schedule: Practice Sun Salutation 5 days a week for 30 minutes, followed by 2 inversion poses, then by Modified Fish Pose and Cool Down. On practice days 1, 3, and 5, follow Modified Fish Pose with Yoga Relief poses. Finish with Cool Down.

Warm Up: Perform Sun Salutation once slowly, holding each posture for 5 breaths.

Sun Salutation: Perform 6 repetitions of Sun Salutation, holding each pose for 1 to 3 breaths.

Inversion Poses—Choose two from the following:

Legs-up-the-wall Pose

Bridge Pose with Strap

Supported Shoulderstand with Wall

Pose of Tranquility

Dolphin Headstand Preparation

Supported Plough Pose

Plus:

Modified Fish Pose (page 168)

Yoga Relief Poses: On practice days 1, 3, and 5, do the 10-Minute Yoga Relief Workout.

Cool Down:

Supported Relaxation Pose

Yoga Relief Poses

YOGA FINGER STRETCH

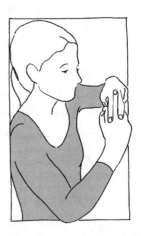

What It Does: Yoga Finger Stretch increases circulation and flexibility in the fingers and hand joints. Be sure to stretch each finger slowly.

How to Do It:

1. Warm up your hands by briskly rubbing them together, as if washing them, for about 10 seconds.

2. Begin by placing the forefinger and middle finger of your left hand on either side of the base of your right thumb. Gently bend back the right thumb.

3. Repeat with each finger of your right hand.

4. Reverse hands and repeat.

YOGA WRIST STRETCH

What It Does: The Yoga Wrist Stretch can help ease strain from repetitive wrist movements, relieve stress in the hands, and increase the flexibility of the wrist.

How to Do It:

1. Warm up your hands and wrists by briskly rubbing them together, as if washing them, for about 10 seconds.

2. Rotate your right wrist to the left in a counterclockwise direction, 5 times. Then rotate it to the right in a clockwise direction, 5 times. Try to keep your right forearm stable throughout, keeping it parallel to the floor.

3. Rotate your left wrist to the right in a clockwise direction, 5 times. Then rotate to the left in counterclockwise direction, 5 times. Try to keep your left forearm stable throughout, keeping it parallel to the floor.

4. With your fingers and palm held gently open, slowly flex and extend your wrists 10 times. Try to maintain a stable forearm throughout, keeping it parallel to the floor.

NAMASTE HAND MUDRA (ANJALI MUDRA)

What It Does: The Namaste Hand Mudra is used as a sacred gesture of greeting, often translated as "The divine in me bows to the divine in you." It is also used to begin Sun Salutation, and with certain postures, such as Mountain Pose or balance poses. Namaste Hand Mudra gently stretches the wrists, hands, and fingers, and helps move crooked fingers back to their normal positions.

How to Do It:

1. Sit on the floor in a cross-legged position, with your spine straight. Drop your chin slightly, extending the back of your neck. If you have difficulty sitting on the floor, or prefer not to do so, you can do this posture by sitting comfortably in a chair with your feet flat on the floor and your shoes off, with your spine straight.

2. Warm up your hands and wrists by briskly rubbing them together, as if washing them, for about 10 seconds.

3. Inhale, slowly drawing your hands together at the center of your

chest in prayer position. If there is wrist pain, bring your forearms together.

4. Exhale as you gently press your fingers and palms together. Press and straighten any crooked fingers. Hold for 2 breaths.

5. Inhale as you gently spread the fingers evenly. Press and straighten any crooked fingers. Hold for 2 breaths.

6. Release the pressure, bringing your fingers back together.

7. As you grow stronger, repeat, gradually increasing the pressure.

YOGA FOOT STRETCH

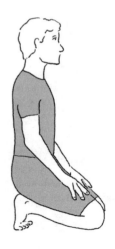

What It Does: Yoga Foot Stretch safely stretches the toes, the ankles, and the soles of the feet. This stretch will also improve the mobility, alignment, and strength of your feet, and relieve tension and pain.

How to Do It:

1. Kneel on the floor with your toes turned under, buttocks resting on your heels and your spine in an upright position. If this pose is difficult to do or painful, try supporting some of your

weight with your hands on the floor. If you still experience pain or discomfort, then stop immediately and come out of this pose.

2. Allow the weight of your body to stretch your toes, feet, and ankles. Hold for 2 full breaths.

3. Release your toes and slowly bring the tops of your feet flat down to the floor. Rest.

4. As you grow stronger and more flexible, repeat the pose.

STAFF POSE (DANDASANA)

What It Does: Doing Staff Pose strengthens the quadriceps muscles (in the front of the thighs), helps stabilize the knees, and keeps the leg bones in proper alignment. It also improves posture and helps prevent a rounded upper back.

How to Do It:

1. Sit on the floor with a folded blanket under your hips and your legs stretched out straight in front of you.

2. Feel the contraction of your quadriceps tendon by placing your

right hand on the bottom edge of your right kneecap. Stretch and straighten your legs, pressing out through your heels. You will feel the right quadriceps tendon tighten and the kneecap will be firm. Repeat this with your left hand to left kneecap. This action stabilizes and strengthens the knee.

3. Now bring your hands flat alongside your hips with your fingers pointing toward your feet. Draw your navel in toward your spine. Stretch and straighten your legs, pressing out through your heels. Contract your quadriceps tendons! Press your shoulders down, away from your ears, and lift your sternum toward the ceiling. Push your palms lightly into the floor. Hold for 2 full breaths.

4. As you grow stronger and more flexible, dispense with the blanket, and repeat the pose.

SALUTE TO GODS AND GODDESSES
(ANJANEYASANA VARIATION)

What It Does: Doing this pose will stretch the quadriceps muscles (in the front of the thighs), as well as tone and strengthen the back, hips, and buttocks.

How to Do It:

1. From a kneeling position, bring your left leg forward, placing your left foot flat on the floor. Place a folded blanket under your right knee for comfort, if necessary. Place your hands on your left knee, maintaining balance.

2. Bring your arms overhead, palms together, thumbs crossed. Inhale, lift, and bend backward, tightening your buttock muscles firmly and tilting your pelvis under, to protect your lower back. Look up. Hold for 1 breath.

3. Slowly come up to starting position, contracting your abdominals. Place your hands on your left knee, maintaining balance.

4. Repeat on the other side.

SIDE ANGLE VARIATION (*PARSVOTTANASANA VARIATION*)

What It Does: Doing Side Angle Variation will safely stretch the hamstrings, help stabilize the knees, and correct poor leg alignment and muscular imbalances.

How to Do It:

1. Place a small table, chair, or stool by your right foot. Stand with your feet 3 to 4 feet apart. Inhale and pivot your right foot out 90 degrees to the right, then pivot your left foot slightly in to the right. Rotate your body to the right to face in the same direction. Tighten the quadriceps and kneecaps.

2. Exhale and bend your torso forward, placing both hands on the stool. Hold for 2 breaths.

3. Inhale, straighten your body up, and return it to center. Repeat on your left side.

YOGA HIP ROCK

What It Does: Yoga Hip Rock will gently stretch your hips, thighs, knees, and ankles and restore to them a greater range of motion. This pose is a good preparation for Half Lotus Pose.

How to Do It:

1. Sit on the floor, with your legs stretched out in front of you. Grasp your right foot and place it inside your left bent elbow. Wrap your right arm around your right knee and clasp your hands together. If you can't keep your left leg stretched in front of you, bend it as much as you need to. With practice you will be able to comfortably stretch into this pose.

2. Sit up tall and relax your shoulders. Now, breathing comfortably, rock your right leg slowly from side to side for 20 to 30 seconds. Feel the stretch around the right hip.

3. Switch legs and repeat on the other side.

BOUND ANGLE POSE *(BADDHA KONASANA)*

What It Does: Bound Angle Pose will gently stretch the hips, thighs, knees, and ankles and restore to them a greater range of motion. This pose is good preparation for Half Lotus Pose.

How to Do It:

1. Sit on the floor, bend your knees, and bring the soles of your feet together. Sit tall, lifting your sternum toward the ceiling. If your spine is rounding, place a folded blanket under your hips.

2. Draw your heels in toward your hips. Place your hands around your feet or your big toes and allow gravity to release your hip joints and pull your knees down toward the floor.

3. Hold for several breaths, breathing comfortably.

HALF LOTUS POSE (ARDHA PADMASANA)

What It Does: Half Lotus Pose is a classic meditation posture that teaches proper leg, ankle, and foot alignment and restores flexibility to the hips and legs. If your hips are very tight, your knees will stick up in the air when you are attempting Half Lotus. If you force this pose, you may cause yourself knee strain. Proceed cautiously and gently. To increase hip flexibility, continue to practice Bound Angle Pose and Yoga Hip Rock for a while before trying Half Lotus Pose again. With practice, your knees will eventually come closer to the floor. You'll find careful, continued practice of Bound Angle, Yoga Hip Rock, and Half Lotus postures to be worthwhile for the long-term health of your hips, knees, ankles, and feet.

How to Do It:

1. Sit on the floor, in a cross-legged position. Gently grasp your right foot and carefully place it as high as possible on top of your left

thigh, with the sole of the foot facing upward. It's okay if you can only get your foot on top of the left inner thigh. The left leg remains in the cross-legged position. Do not force this position! If your right knee feels strain or pain, or is sticking up in the air, you're not ready to do this pose.

2. Sit up straight, lifting your sternum, your palms resting on your knees. Hold for a few seconds, breathing comfortably.

3. Gently release the right foot back to cross-legged position. Repeat the pose with your left foot.

MODIFIED WARRIOR I
(*MODIFIED VIRABHADRASANA I*)

What It Does: Warrior I strengthens the legs and hips and improves balance and stamina. As its name implies, this is a pose of power and strength. When you feel comfortable and strong doing Warrior I without the aid of a wall, practice Warrior II.

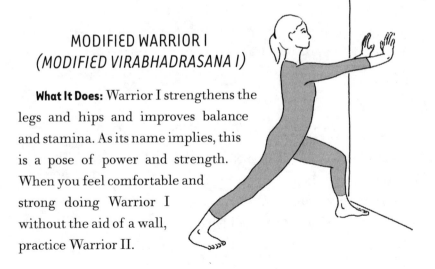

How to Do It:

1. Place your hands on the wall shoulder-width apart and a little above shoulder height. Stand with your feet 3 to 4 feet apart, the left foot facing forward with toes touching the wall and the right foot turned out.

2. Bend your left leg until it is close to a right angle. The right leg is straight. Square your hips to face the wall. Press your shoulder blades down as you push against the wall with your hands.

3. Inhale and straighten your left leg, keeping your hands against the wall. Exhale and bend the left leg. Repeat 2 times.

4. Repeat the pose on the other side. When you no longer need the wall for support, raise both arms over your head with your palms facing each other.

WARRIOR II (*VIRABHADRASANA II*)

What It Does: Warrior II stretches and strengthens the muscles that support the knees, including the quadriceps and hamstrings. You are ready to practice Warrior II when you feel comfortable and strong doing Warrior I without the wall for support.

How to Do It:

1. Inhale and step your feet about 4 feet apart, then pivot your right foot 90 degrees out to the right. Pivot your left foot slightly in, approximately 15 degrees, toward the right side. Extend your arms out to the sides in line with your shoulders, your palms facing down.

2. Exhale and bend your right knee until it's directly over your right ankle, forming a right angle. If you are not able to form the right angle initially, cautiously bend your right knee as far as you can comfortably go while still maintaining control and alignment. Don't let your knee roll in or out, or extend beyond the ankle. Turn your head to look toward the extended fingertips of your right hand.

3. Straighten your legs and repeat on the opposite side.

HERO POSE (*VIRASANA*)

What It Does: Hero Pose stretches the quadriceps muscles, knees, ankles, and tops of the feet. Start by sitting with a folded blanket, a book, or a block under your hips. Gradually lower the prop as you become more flexible, until you can sit comfortably on the floor between your feet without one.

How to Do It:

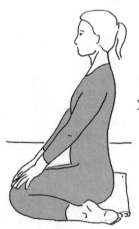

1. Kneel on the floor with your shin bones pointing straight back and parallel to each other, and the tops of your feet extended and pointing straight back. Keep your spine in an upright position. Be sure to have your shins and feet in correct alignment, or you will strain your knees. Sit on a folded blanket or a telephone book placed between your feet. Rest your palms on your knees. Feel the stretch at the tops of your thighs, and in your ankles and feet. Rest your palms on your knees. Breathe and hold for a few seconds.

2. When you're ready, lower or remove the prop—but don't force anything! If your knees, ankles, or feet feel strain or pain, stop!

3. To come out of the pose, return to kneeling.

EAGLE POSE (GARUDASANA)

What It Does: Eagle Pose stretches the shoulder blades, arms, and hands; strengthens the legs; and improves balance and stamina. Practice the arm and leg sequences separately until you can maintain control, alignment, and balance. Stand near a chair or wall for support, if necessary.

How to Do It:

1. Practice Eagle arms first. Begin in Mountain Pose (see page 26). Bend your right elbow and raise it to chest level. Cross your left arm and elbow under your right upper arm and elbow. Join your palms together. Feel the stretch across your shoulders and upper back. Breathe softly and hold.

2. Repeat on the opposite side, reversing the cross of the arms.

3. Now practice Eagle legs. Begin in Mountain Pose. Stand near a chair or wall for support. Bend your left knee, then cross and wrap your right leg over your left thigh and hook your right ankle around the back of your left ankle. If you have difficulty hooking the right ankle behind the left ankle, simply lower your right foot so the tops of the toes rest on the floor. Breathe softly and balance for a few seconds. Release and return to Mountain Pose.

4. Repeat on the opposite side, reversing the cross of the legs.

5. When you feel you can maintain control, alignment, and balance, combine the Eagle arm and leg sequences. Begin in Mountain Pose. Cross your left arm and elbow under your right upper arm and elbow. Join your palms together. Bend your left knee, then cross and wrap your right leg over your left thigh and hook your right ankle around the back of your left ankle. If you have difficulty hooking the right ankle behind the left ankle, simply lower your right foot so the tops of the toes rest on the floor. Breathe and balance!

7. Repeat on the opposite side, reversing the cross of the arms and legs.

PRANA BREATHING *(PRANAYAMA VARIATION)*

What It Does: Prana Breathing increases prana (the life-force energy), facilitates healing, and relieves stress. It releases tension and stretches the shoulder blades, arms, and hands. It also stimulates acupressure points between the shoulder blades, revitalizing the respiratory, circulatory, and nervous systems.

How to Do It:

1. Stand straight. Inhale slowly through your nose and spread your arms out to your sides. The palms are facing forward. Feel your breath expanding from the center of your chest out through your arms, to the tips of your fingers. Continue expanding your arms backward, keeping them straight, opening your chest, gently squeezing your shoulder blades together, and bringing your head back. Expand the feeling of the breath through your body, down to your toes.

2. Exhale slowly through your nose and bring your arms forward, palms meeting in front of

you, as you curve your spine inward and bring your head forward. Bring the expansive feeling back to the center of your chest.

3. Continue Prana Breathing slowly and rhythmically, opening and closing your arms and body with each breath. Continue for 30 to 60 seconds.

chapter 7

Yoga for Sex and Vitality

Yoga for Lifelong Vitality

You can enjoy middle age and continue to live a healthy, youthful life well into your golden years by practicing the revitalizing yoga workout that follows. You may be one of the millions of baby boomers who now are approaching or in the midst of their middle years, and experiencing perimenopause, menopause, osteoporosis, prostate problems, diminished sexual drive, or impotence. With regular practice, these simple, effective yoga postures can ease many of the uncomfortable symptoms associated with this time of life and open the way to embracing, honoring, and even celebrating it as a period of change and personal growth.

Approximately seventy-six million baby boomers, more men and women born than at any other time in the history of the United States, will be experiencing midlife and menopause at the same time.

This unprecedented demographic shift is bound to create profound social, economic, and cultural changes. Hopefully a more enlightened approach to and view of menopause and midlife will also emerge. Historically, this phase of life was considered a transition into old age, but that view no longer holds true. Advances in medicine and health combined with changes in attitudes have given twenty-first-century baby boomers confidence that they still have a lot of living to do. Since the average age of menopause is fifty and life expectancy has lengthened, boomers can anticipate living from one-third to half their lives after menopause and middle age.

Many midlife changes, such as diminishing hormone levels, weight gain, and loss of libido, can be alleviated by embracing healthy lifestyle changes, like the practice of yoga. Doing yoga helps to balance the endocrine system and evens out the hormonal changes of midlife. Yoga's weight-bearing poses strengthen bones and help prevent osteoporosis. Specific yoga postures increase circulation to the reproductive organs and the prostate, thereby contributing to a healthy, active, Viagra-free sex life.

As the first wave of the baby boom generation begins the journey into midlife and menopause, yoga can become an important cornerstone of lifelong health.

Yoga and "the Change"

Menopause, or "the change of life," marks the end of a woman's fertility, the cessation of ovulation and menstruation. The hormonal changes of menopause can create a barrage of symptoms, including hot flashes, night sweats, mood swings, diminished sexual desire, heart palpitations, hair loss on the scalp and hair growth on the face, weight gain, and bone demineralization leading to osteoporosis. These physical changes were once treated by the medical profession and our society as manifestations of a disease or a deficiency. Happily, attitudes are changing. Menopause is now viewed as a normal event, a natural transition from the childbearing years to later life. Many women have come to celebrate menopause as a time of wisdom, personal empowerment, and newfound sexual freedom.

The first step in "the change" occurs with perimenopause, a transitional stage that can last for ten or more years before actual menopause begins. Women in their mid to late thirties and early forties may experience irregular hormone levels and PMS-like symptoms, such as bloating, difficulty in sleeping, mood swings, and breast tenderness.

Research has shown that exercise, including the yoga practice described here, can help to ease the uncomfortable symptoms that accompany perimenopause and menopause. You can reduce the incidence of hot flashes and night sweats with cooling yoga poses that place the head below the heart, such as One-Legged Downward-Facing Dog, Modified Peacock Pose, and Legs-up-the Wall Pose. Other poses, such as Yoga Squat, Half Lord of the Fishes Pose, Bow Pose, and Modified Fish Pose, improve balance, relieve hormonal and vaginal changes, increase circulation to the thyroid and adrenal glands, and tone the abdomen, pelvis, and reproductive organs.

Building Strong Bones

You may not be particularly concerned about osteoporosis because you mistakenly believe that it is a problem exclusive to frail, elderly women. Although osteoporosis has traditionally been associated with older women, it is a disease that can begin at a relatively young age and can affect otherwise healthy men and women. "Osteoporosis" is defined as a loss of bone mass, specifically when the body loses more bone cells than it creates. As you might imagine, this decrease in bone density leads to bone fragility and an increased risk of fractures.

Your bones, which seem so solid and static, are actually living, growing tissue. During childhood, more bone is made than lost. Our bone mass reaches its peak density level at around age thirty. Peak bone density depends to some extent on how much calcium and other nutrients you absorbed during childhood. Building strong bones during childhood and adolescence can be the best way to prevent osteoporosis. However, due to poor nutrition, genetics, and other factors, many youngsters do not build up sufficient bone mass to withstand later losses. By around age forty, both men and women begin a slow, age-related bone loss.

For women, this bone loss speeds up after menopause, when estrogen levels decline. According to the National Osteoporosis Foundation, twenty-eight million Americans, 80 percent of them women, are affected by osteoporosis. The National Osteoporosis Foundation warns that a woman's chance of suffering a hip fracture is equal to her combined risk of contracting breast, uterine, and ovarian cancer. One in two women and one in eight men over age fifty will have an osteoporosis-related fracture in their lifetime, resulting in more than 1.5 million bone fractures each year.

Osteoporosis isn't only a woman's disease; over two million American men have this "silent disease" as well. Although men don't experience the sudden speeding up of bone loss that women undergo after menopause, by age sixty-five, men and women lose bone at the same rate. Many people don't realize that they have osteoporosis because it often isn't diagnosed until a relatively minor accident causes a fracture. A bone density test (also called a BMD, or bone mineral density, test) can detect osteoporosis before a fracture occurs; it can also be used to determine your rate of bone loss and monitor the effects of treatment. Consult your physician to determine whether you should have a BMD test.

Although it's ideal to begin osteoporosis prevention before the age of thirty, the good news is, it's never too late to prevent further bone loss. The best way to do so is with lifestyle changes that build strong bones, such as eating a balanced diet rich in calcium and vitamin D and regular practice of weight-bearing exercise. Most experts recommend a half hour of weight-bearing exercise (such as yoga, weight lifting, or walking) daily. Yoga postures stimulate your bones to retain calcium through the bearing of weight by the legs and arms. This combats bone loss by placing stress on the bones, which in turn encourages new bone growth. Yoga practice also improves balance, posture, and body mechanics, thus decreasing the likelihood of a traumatic fall or fractures. For example, standing yoga postures, such as Revolved Triangle Pose, Modified Half Moon Pose, and Warrior III Preparation, can improve balance, coordination, and body mechanics, which can help to prevent potential falls and fractures. Inverted weight-bearing yoga postures, such as One-Legged Downward-Facing Dog and Modified Peacock Pose, strengthen bones in the upper and lower body.

Yoga for Men

Menopause doesn't affect only women. Middle-aged men often complain of or suffer from weight gain, loss of sexual interest, muscle and bone loss, depression, and lack of energy. The symptoms of "male menopause," known as andropause or viropause, can result from decreased hormone levels due to aging as well as unhealthy lifestyle habits. According to experts, these symptoms can be prevented and reversed by lifestyle changes that include regular exercise and, in certain situations, testosterone therapy.

Many middle-age men also begin experiencing an increased urge to urinate. Benign prostate enlargement, or benign prostatic hyperplasia (BPH), is often the cause. In BPH, the prostate slowly enlarges, leading to increased urinary frequency or other difficulties with urination. Urinary problems can also be a sign of prostate cancer, the most common cancer in American men except for skin cancer. For this reason, the American Cancer Society recommends annual PSA (prostate-specific antigen) tests and DRE (digital rectal exam) for all men fifty and over, to help detect the presence of cancer. Research shows that positive lifestyle changes, including a healthy diet and regular exercise, can help prevent prostate problems.

The yoga workout program in this chapter can help men sail smoothly through andropause and avoid prostate problems. Yoga poses such as Bow Pose, Half Lord of the Fishes Pose, Yoga Sitting Cat, and Lying Bound Angle Pose tone the abdomen, pelvis, and reproductive organs; balance hormones; and promote circulation to the prostate gland. Yoga mula bandha, or "root lock," which contracts the perineum, will help strengthen the urinary sphincter and benefit the urogenital tract.

Yoga and Sexuality

Some people—generally those under thirty!—have the mistaken impression that menopause means the end of their sexuality. The pleasant and exciting truth is that midlife marks the middle of active sex life as well. Both women and men can have gratifying sex after menopause/andropause and feel wonderful about themselves.

Sexual problems do occur but often can be remedied. Impotence has many causes, such as testosterone deficiency, libido-lowering medications, disease, stress, or injury. Counseling is often recommended if there is a psychological issue, such as performance anxiety or marital dissatisfaction. However, in many cases the underlying problem is due to a less-than-healthy lifestyle. Impotence may be prevented by positive lifestyle changes, including a healthy diet and regular exercise.

Increasing your flexibility with yoga practice means more sexual positions will be available to you. Yoga poses such as Lying Bound Angle Pose and Yoga Squat can be done by men and women to increase flexibility and promote circulation through the pelvis and reproductive organs.

Tantric yoga practice can help enhance everyone's sexuality. Tantric sacred sexuality has recently been reintroduced and popularized in the United States. This branch of yoga seeks balance, inner peace, and transcendence through everyday acts of life such as eating, breathing, and the sacred union of the male and female.

The ancient precepts of tantra yoga, written almost two thousand years ago, can be very useful in helping to heal sexual dysfunctions.

An essential tantric yoga pose, mula bandha, or "root lock," offers many health benefits to men and women. Mula bandha is similar to Kegel exercises, which train and strengthen the muscles of the pelvic floor, increase sexual pleasure, reduce incontinence, improve the health of the prostate, and slow the aging of the perineum. Other tantric poses, such as Yoga Sitting Cat and Yoga Standing Cat, promote circulation through the pelvis and reproductive organs, strengthen the sexual system, and raise sexual energy.

Before You Start

- Keep in mind that if you're just beginning a fitness program, you should comfortably and gradually work up to the suggested frequency and duration of the poses.
- Perform the poses slowly and consciously, according to your abilities. You should never be in pain, and there should not be a feeling of breathlessness. If you feel discomfort, stop and come out of the pose.

- Always consult your physician before beginning a new exercise program.

Yoga for Sexual Vitality Workout

If your time is limited, the Yoga for Sexual Vitality Workout can be practiced on its own. You will reap benefits even if you have only 10 minutes to do this yoga practice. For maximum longevity benefits, combine this workout with any of the Yoga Fountain of Youth Workouts in Chapter 4. For example, see the combination of the Maintenance Fountain of Youth Workout and the Yoga for Sexual Vitality Workout that follows.

Be aware that it may take you more than 4 weeks to do this routine comfortably, depending on your physical condition. If you feel comfortable and confident doing the poses in Weeks 1 and 2, proceed to Weeks 3 and 4. Otherwise, stay with Weeks 1 and 2 until you feel strong enough to continue.

Weeks 1 and 2

Practice Schedule: Practice for 10 to 15 minutes, 3 days a week. For each workout, choose at least two gender-appropriate poses, then follow with at least one additional pose for Sexual Vitality.

Poses for Women—Choose at least two from the following:

Bow Pose

Modified Fish Pose

Warrior III Preparation

Poses for Men—Choose at least two from the following:

Bow Pose

Modified Fish Pose

Half Lord of the Fishes Pose

Poses for Sexual Vitality—Choose at least one from the following:

Mula Bandha (page 30)

Yoga Sitting Cat

Lying Bound Angle Pose

Weeks 3 and 4

Practice Schedule: Practice for 10 to 15 minutes, 3 days a week. For each workout, choose at least two gender-appropriate poses, then follow with at least one additional pose for Sexual Vitality.

Poses for Women—Choose at least two from the following:

Modified Half Moon Pose

Revolved Triangle Pose

One-Legged Downward-Facing Dog

Peacock Pose Preparation

Poses for Men—Choose at least two from the following:

Lying Bound Angle Pose

Modified Half Moon Pose

Revolved Triangle Pose

Poses for Sexual Vitality—Choose at least one from the following:

Half Lord of the Fishes Pose

Yoga Standing Cat

Yoga Squat

Maintenance Fountain of Youth and Yoga for Sexual Vitality Workout

A combination of the 10-minute Yoga for Sexual Vitality Workout and the Maintenance Fountain of Youth Workout will help ease midlife changes and increase sexual vitality, as well as build and maintain your cardiovascular fitness, strength, and flexibility.

Week 1 and Beyond

Workout Schedule: Practice Sun Salutation 5 days a week for 30 minutes, followed by 2 inversion poses, plus Modified Fish Pose and Cool

Down. On practice days 1, 3, and 5, follow Modified Fish Pose with the Yoga for Sexual Vitality Workout. Finish with Cool Down.

Warm Up: Perform Sun Salutation once slowly, holding each posture for 5 breaths.

Sun Salutation: Perform 6 repetitions of Sun Salutation, holding each pose for 1 to 3 breaths.

Inversion Poses—Choose two from the following:

Legs-up-the-Wall Pose

Bridge Pose with Strap

Supported Shoulderstand with Wall

Pose of Tranquility

Dolphin Headstand Preparation

Supported Plough Pose

Plus:

Modified Fish Pose

Yoga for Sexual Vitality Workout: On practice days 1, 3, and 5, do the poses for 10 to 15 minutes.

Cool Down:

Supported Relaxation Pose

Yoga for Sexual Vitality Poses

MODIFIED HALF MOON POSE
(MODIFIED ARDHA CHANDRASANA)

What It Does: The Modified Half Moon Pose is a weight-bearing standing pose that if done correctly stimulates the bones of the arms, legs, and spine to retain calcium. Practice this pose against a wall for added stability and use a block or prop under your hand to help you maintain proper alignment, especially if you are stiff or weak. As you grow more flexible, balanced, and confident, dispense with the block and practice with only the wall for additional support.

How to Do It:

1. Stand straight, with your back to the wall, your buttocks lightly touching it, and your feet 3 to 4 feet apart. Pivot your left foot 90 degrees to the right and then your right foot 30 degrees inward.

2. Inhale and bring your

arms out to the sides in a T position. Exhale and glide your torso to the left, bending your left knee in order to place the fingertips of your left hand on the floor or on a block placed approximately 12 inches beyond the toes of your left foot.

3. Inhale and shift the weight onto your left leg, straightening your left leg as your raise your right leg to the level of your pelvis. Exhale and push strongly through the right heel while lifting the right hip toward the ceiling and drawing it toward the wall. Look forward and extend your right arm up toward the ceiling. Breathe and hold the pose for 30 seconds.

4. To release, bend your left leg and slowly lower your right foot to the floor, returning to standing position.

5. Repeat the pose on the opposite side.

REVOLVED TRIANGLE POSE *(PARIVARTTA TRIKONASANA)*

What It Does: Revolved Triangle is a combination of a forward bend, a twist, and a weight-bearing standing pose. It stimulates the bones of the arms, legs, and spine to retain calcium, which is essential in building bone mass to combat osteoporosis. Practice this more advanced posture when you feel comfortable and strong doing Standing Forward Bend (see page 75). Use a chair or block to help you maintain proper alignment, especially if you are stiff or weak. As you grow more flexible, balanced, and confident, try practicing this pose without the prop. Individuals with disc injuries should not practice this or other twisting poses without the assistance of an experienced teacher.

How to Do It:

1. Assume a wide stance, feet 3 to 4 feet apart, arms out to the sides in a T position. Pivot your left foot 90 degrees to the left and your right foot 30 degrees to the left, so that your left heel is in line with the arch of your right foot. Square your hips to face your left foot.

2. Exhale, rotating your torso and bending forward, and resting

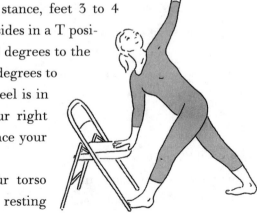

the fingertips of your right hand on the outside of your left foot. Stretch your left arm overhead. Pull your abdomen in. If it is comfortable to do so, turn your head to look up. (If you can't reach the floor, rest your right hand on a chair or block.)

3. Keep reaching, lifting, and lengthening as you hold the pose for 3 or 4 breaths.

4. Straighten up and repeat on the other side.

ONE-LEGGED DOWNWARD-FACING DOG
(ADHO MUKHA SVANASANA VARIATION)

What It Does: One-Legged Downward-Facing Dog is an inverted weight-bearing pose that places the head below the heart, helping to reduce the incidence of hot flashes and night sweats. Properly practiced, it can strengthen the bones in the upper and lower body.

How to Do It:

1. Begin on your hands and knees, with your hands directly below your shoulders

and your knees below your hips. Exhale, lifting your hips as you turn your body into an upside-down V. Keep your arms and legs straight and press your heels into the floor. Press your shoulders down, away from your ears.

2. Inhale and extend your left leg up toward the ceiling in line with your back, and press your right heel toward the floor. Exhale and bring your left leg back to the floor.

3. Repeat with the right leg.

BOW POSE (DHANURASANA)

What It Does: Doing the Bow Pose properly can help to balance and relieve hormonal and vaginal changes; increase circulation to the thyroid, adrenal glands, and prostate; and tone the abdomen, pelvis, and reproductive organs and glands.

How to Do It:

1. Lie on your stomach with your forehead on the mat. Reach back and grasp your ankles firmly, keeping your knees hip-width apart. The arms are straight.

2. Inhale, then exhale, lifting your forehead, nose, and chin. Raise your chest off the floor. To protect your lower back, tighten your buttocks and tuck your pelvis under. Raise your knees off the floor.

3. Inhale, squeeze your shoulder blades together, and lift your breastbone up. Relax your neck.

4. Exhale, releasing the intensity of the stretch slightly, then inhale, lifting your chest and rib cage a little further.

5. Hold for a moment. Exhale and release the stretch slightly, then inhale and lift the chest even higher.

6. Release hands from ankles and lie on your stomach. Rest for a moment.

7. Repeat.

WARRIOR III PREPARATION
(VIRABHADRASANA III PREPARATION)

What It Does: Doing Warrior III Preparation stimulates the bones of the arms, legs, and spine to retain calcium, which is essential in building bone mass to combat osteoporosis. This pose is practiced in an all-fours tabletop position in preparation for Modified Warrior III (see page 52).

How to Do It:

1. Begin on hands and knees, with your back flat like a tabletop. Inhale and shift your weight onto your right arm while raising your left arm straight forward. Look downward. Exhale and hold the position.

2. Repeat the action on your other side.

3. Inhale and shift your weight onto your left leg, while straigthen-

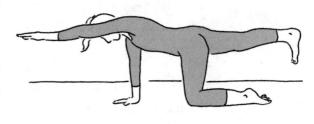

ing and raising your right leg. Exhale and hold, pushing through the right heel.

4. Repeat the action on the other side.

5. Now combine the two actions. From tabletop position, inhale and shift your weight onto your right arm while straightening and raising your left arm, and shift your weight onto your left leg while raising your right leg. Exhale and hold.

6. Repeat, changing sides.

MODIFIED FISH POSE (MODIFIED MATSYASANA)

What It Does: Modified Fish Pose can increase circulation to your thyroid, adrenal glands, and lymph nodes, and can help your posture 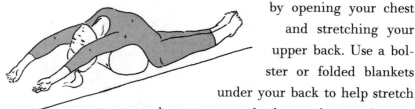 by opening your chest and stretching your upper back. Use a bolster or folded blankets under your back to help stretch and open your neck, throat, chest, and upper back. Fish Pose should always follow shoulderstands (see Supported Shoulderstand with Wall, page 80).

How to Do It:

1. Sit with your legs straight in front of you and the small of your back a few inches away from a bolster. Then lean against the bolster and arch your back over it. Slowly drop your head back. Keep your arms straight at your sides. Take 2 deep breaths.

2. Raise your arms toward the ceiling and gently move them behind your head, so the backs of your hands touch the floor. Bend your arms if you are stiff and you find this action painful. Taking full, deep breaths, hold the pose for up to a minute.

3. To come out of the pose, roll to one side, then use your arms to help you sit up.

PEACOCK POSE PREPARATION
(PINCHA MAYURASANA PREPARATION)

What It Does: Peacock Pose Preparation is an inverted weight-bearing pose that places the head below the heart, helping to reduce the incidence of hot flashes and night sweats. Doing this pose properly can strengthen bones in the upper and lower body.

How to Do It:

1. Kneel on the floor, then rest your forearms and palms on the mat in front of you, elbows directly below your shoulders. Measure the distance between your elbows by placing your left fist against your right elbow.

2. Exhale as you lift your hips, straightening your knees. The balls of the feet, forearms, and palms press firmly into the mat. Draw your shoulders away from your ears and draw

your chest back toward your thighs. Hold the pose for up to a minute, taking calm, even breaths.

4. To come out of the pose, lower your knees to the mat into a kneeling position. Keep your head down for a few moments before sitting up.

HALF LORD OF THE FISHES POSE *(ARDHA MATSYENDRASANA)*

What It Does: Half Lord of the Fishes tones the abdomen, pelvis, and reproductive organs, balances the hormones, and promotes circulation to the prostate gland.

How to Do It:

1. Begin by kneeling, buttocks resting on the backs of your heels. Place your left hand on the floor and gently shift your weight down to the left until you are sitting to the left of your feet, keeping your legs bent under you. Cross your right leg over your left knee, so that the right foot is flat on the floor alongside the left knee

and the left foot is resting against the back of the right thigh. Then place the fingertips of your right hand on the floor, behind your right buttock. Inhale.

2. Exhale, then twist your torso and place your left arm and elbow against your outer right lower thigh. Bend your left arm, pressing it against the right lower thigh, with your left fingertips pointed toward the ceiling. Gaze over your right shoulder.

3. Inhale and lengthen your spine. Exhale and deepen the twist to the right. Hold the pose for several breaths.

4. Release the twist and repeat on the other side.

LYING BOUND ANGLE POSE *(SUPTA BADDHA KONASANA)*

What It Does: Lying Bound Angle Pose promotes circulation to the pelvis, reproductive organs, and prostate gland and balances the hormones. Use a bolster or two folded blankets under your back, a folded blanket under your head, and a folded blanket under your thighs, to help stretch and open your pelvis, groin, and hips.

How to Do It:

1. Sit on the floor in front of the blankets and bring the soles of your feet together. Lie back, keeping your soles together, until your head is resting on the blankets, with your back, neck, and head fully supported, and your arms open, your hands palms-up.

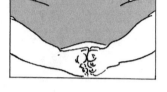

2. Close your eyes; relax your face, throat, and groin; and take calm breaths through your nose. Rest in this pose for up to 5 minutes.

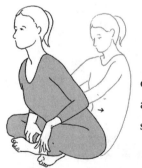

YOGA SITTING CAT
(CHAKRAVAKASANA VARIATION 2)

What It Does: Yoga Sitting Cat tones the abdomen, promotes circulation through the pelvis and reproductive organs, strengthens the sexual system, and raises sexual energy and endurance.

How to Do It:

1. Sit on the floor with your legs crossed and your hands holding your shins.

2. Inhale as you press your torso forward, lifting your chest and

sternum. Think about lengthening the front of your body. Keep your shoulders down, away from your ears.

3. Exhale and in a flowing motion return your spine to an upright position; then round your back like a cat. Pull your stomach up and in toward your spine and look down at the floor. Hold. Release.

4. Repeat, establishing a smooth transition—inhaling as your torso moves forward, exhaling as you round your back. Repeat 10 times.

YOGA STANDING CAT (*CHAKRAVAKASANA VARIATION #3*)

What It Does: Yoga Standing Cat tones the abdomen, promotes circulation through the pelvis and reproductive organs, releases tension, strengthens the sexual and hormonal systems, and raises sexual energy and endurance.

How to Do It:

1. Stand with your back straight, feet hip-width apart, knees slightly bent, and hands resting on your knees.

2. Inhale as you press your torso forward and lift your chest, sternum, and chin, lengthening the front of your body and arching your lower back.

3. Exhale and in a flowing motion return your spine to an

upright position; then round your back like a cat. Pull your stomach up and in toward your spine and look down at the floor. Hold. Release, relaxing your spine and abdomen.

4. Establish a smooth flow of inhaling while arching your lower back, and exhaling while rounding the back. Repeat 10 times.

YOGA SQUAT (MALASANA)

What It Does: Doing the Yoga Squat properly can promote circulation through the pelvis and reproductive organs and increase the flexibility of the lower back, pelvis, hips, and legs.

How to Do It:

1. Stand with your feet slightly wider than hip-width apart, pointed straight ahead. Do not point your feet out or in, as this will strain your knees. Squat comfortably down on your heels, with your arms resting on your knees.

2. Breathe deeply as you drop your tailbone and lift your chest and sternum. Hold for up to a minute.

3. To come out of the pose, press down through your feet and rise with the strength of your thighs, continuing to lift through the torso.

Index

About the Author

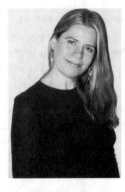

ELAINE GAVALAS received her master's degree from Columbia University in New York. She's an exercise physiologist, health expert, and weight management specialist who works with groups and individuals of all sizes, shapes, and ages to help them reach and maintain their ideal weight, wellness, and fitness goals. She utilizes yoga and fitness techniques that integrate the body, mind, and spirit.

Her yoga minibook series includes *The Yoga Minibook for Weight Loss, The Yoga Minibook for Stress Relief, The Yoga Minibook for Longevity,* and *The Yoga Minibook for Energy and Strength.* Gavalas is the author of numerous yoga, fitness, and diet articles and books, including *Secrets of Fat-Free Greek Cooking* (1998).

If you or your company would like to contact Elaine or want more information about her books, videotapes, or group and individual services, visit her website at www.yogaminibooks.com or e-mail her at AskElaineG @aol.com.

Exercise your body, soul, and mind with the entire series of Yoga Minibooks

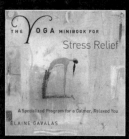

The Yoga Minibook for Stress Relief

0-7432-2701-8 · $10.00

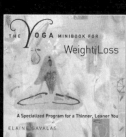

The Yoga Minibook for Weight Loss

0-7432-2698-4 · $10.00

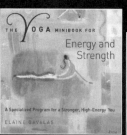

The Yoga Minibook for Energy and Strength

0-7432-2700-X · $10.00

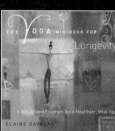

The Yoga Minibook for Longevity

0-7432-2699-2 · $10.00

FIRESIDE
A Division of Simon & Schuster
A VIACOM COMPANY